Table of Contents

Acknowledgments

Thanks to Marilyn Wann, Linda Bacon, Deb Burgard, & Jon Robison, and those who have been on the front lines since the early days who I have not yet met. Your tireless work does not go unnoticed. I admire you, I appreciate you, and I thank you.

Thanks to CJ Legare, Golda Poretsky, Kath Read, Dr. Deah, Jennifer Jonassen, Virginia Sole-Smith, Susie Klein, Jayne Williams, Rebecca Weinstein, the Fierce Fatties, Jay and Eszter Solomon, Kelly Bliss, and everyone I'm forgetting in the pressure of this moment– your work is a lifeline to me!

Thanks to my publicist Karin Maake of Blueprint PR, I have no idea how you put up with me, but I'm very glad that you do!

Thanks to my get-shit-done-soulmate Jeanette DePatie for mad tech skills, help with this book, and just being awesome.

Thanks to Julianne and the Los Angeles Fat Mafia for being inspiring, supportive, hilarious, and amazing all at the same time.

Thanks to Mark Land and David Jones – you are lunch time geniuses.

Thanks to Darryl Roberts for your work, your openness, and being brave enough to put me in, and keep me in, your film.

Thanks to Kathy, Kelly, Maria, Jeanette, and Nina for reading this when it was a mess and giving crucial feedback.

Thanks to my blog Members, your support means the world to me and made this book possible.

Huge Massive Special Thanks to all of my blog readers, Twitter followers, and Facebook friends whose inspire me every day. I love you guys!

Dedication

To My Mom: No offense to all of the other moms out there, but my Mom, Michele Lutz, is the best Mom in the whole wide world. Her unending, unshakeable, support of me and my dreams started before I was born and continues to this day. For every time you sat in the principal's office and defended me, for every time you fought beside me for something that I wanted to do that someone said was impossible, for every time you took my phone call and listened to me and offered to get on a plane to give me a hug, for letting me tell funny stories about you in the blog and on stand-up stages, for all of your support and everything that you are, I will never be able to thank you enough. I would not be the person I am today without you. I love you to bunches and bunches and lots and lots to infinity to the power of infinity squared.

To Kelrick Drake-Sargent, my Best Friend and adopted brother. What do you say to the person who spent 5 hours ironing your wedding dress even though he knew you were making a huge mistake? What do you say to the person who always has a space for you in his world, who knows all of your secrets and tells you his, who tells you the truth, who spent a day watching every showing of the Lion King at Disney World? Thank you doesn't seem like enough, but it's what I've got. Thank you!

To Kenny Drake-Sargent, the newest addition to the family. Thank you for your patience, your understanding, your friendship, your patience, welcoming me into your home, your cooking, your counsel, your patience, and did I mention your patience? You are an amazing person and I'm so happy to have you in my life. Thank you!

Foreword by Marilyn Wann

First, let me tell you this is a thoroughly fabulous book for people of all sizes, for anyone who's ever felt even a momentary twinge of unhappiness about weight. If you're eager to read about fun attitude and awesome information, just skip my comments here and go ahead and start reading the brilliant essays Ragen has assembled for you.

If you're like me, and you sometimes (often) put off experiences that are likely to be wholly good, I have a confession: I've been putting off writing this foreword. It's not about laziness or lack of motivation, it's about fear. In this case, fear that I'm not good enough to speak on behalf of such a good book and such a good friend and activist, with perhaps some fear that whatever I write will not be good enough to express how good this book is and how much I think you will love it, too.

This fear of not being good enough stops a lot of us from enjoying good things in life. Combine that with a totally rational and justified fear of being judged and treated badly for what we weigh, and it's so easy to miss so many good things in life that it amounts to missing out on life itself. That is crushingly sad and painful and wrong.

There's a way out of this society-created/self-created trap. It does not require you to become perfect, to lose weight, to have an invincibly positive attitude, or to know everything. It's about fabulousness.

Fabulousness, for me, is code for that thing human beings can do in the face of unfairness and injustice and fear, when we say, "Hell, no, I'm not taking it any more!" and we do something...fabulous...to change the situation. But the situation starts to change before we do anything at all. It starts to change in that moment when we turn away from fear (which can, admittedly, be very attention-grabbing!) and we turn toward fabulousness (which, I promise, can be equally beguiling, but way more fun!). Fabulousness doesn't make you perfect, thin, or all-knowing, it makes you better than these categories, just as you are. Fabulousness is not something you need to find; it's an option you already have at any moment, even the worst moments.

What has just helped me stop putting off the blissful honor of writing a foreword for this book is remembering that my fear is nowhere near as strong as fabulousness. Leaping into fabulousness is what Ragen Chastain does all the time, in her life as a proud, health-seeking, prejudice-thwarting fat person and in her writing on these topics. As you read this book, you'll take in all sorts of attitude and information and they'll be life-changing and revolutionary in themselves, but remember also to notice how these quick-read, hard- hitting, awe-inspiring essays from Ragen also play a constant backbeat of turning fear into fabulousness.

When the bullies and hatemongers come at you for what you weigh (whatever you happen to weigh!), they are attempting to install fear in you. They're certainly not being helpful! It feels wrong. It hurts.
It can really stay with a person, being bullied or excluded or treated badly or just plain never welcomed warmly...for who we are. Like I said, plenty of justified reasons for fear. But also even more reasons for fabulousness.

I mention attitude and information because I have noticed both in myself and in other people, that when we contemplate disagreeing with weight hate, we want reliable, protective tools to help us; often, the tools that reassure us are positive attitude and a big supply of impressive information. These tools are super useful for fighting the good fights: "Look, I don't feel the way you feel! Here's why I think differently, too!" You will find all sorts of great attitude and information in this book. Make them your own, rely on them, and use them as much as you like! But also, remember that if you happen not to feel that empowered attitude in a particular moment, if you happen to forget the conclusive information that would counter some piece of weight hate, you're still okay. You don't need to give up hope and start putting off all the good things in life. You don't need to feel inadequate or unworthy. You don't need to fear. Because you're fabulous. No reason. You just are.

~Marilyn

Prologue

Why An Owner's Manual?

As a fat person in Western Culture, I am acutely aware that a war is being fought against me. As a trained researcher who has spent countless hours poring over research I know what we are being told about weight and health is not what is reflected in the evidence.

It's never my goal to tell people how to live, only to make sure people have good information and are aware of all of their options. This book is about doing exactly that. Whether you want to lose weight, fight for size acceptance, or just live your best life I wanted to write a book that would help you navigate our culture in the body you have now, make decisions for your future, and examine the culture that makes a book like this necessary.

If you're a fellow fatty, then welcome; I'm very happy to be in the living life in the fat lane with you!

If you aren't fat and you're reading this book to gain better understanding and/or support your fat friends and family, thank you from the bottom of my big fat heart. When you're fat in this culture, sometimes it can feel like the whole world thinks you are lazy, unhealthy and unattractive. So it is always awesome to know there are people in the world who get it.

I wrote this book as a way to research and answer some questions that I had, like:

Why is it accepted that some people who eat a ton of food stay thin but not accepted that some people who eat a small amount of food stay fat?

Since many thin people get diabetes, heart disease and high blood pressure, why is becoming thin suggested as a cure or preventative?

Why do we use BMI as a measure for metabolic health when we can easily and accurately test metabolic health measures directly?

Since doctors treat joint pain in thin people with options other than weight loss, why don't they give fat people those same treatments?

Why do we believe doing unhealthy things (liquid diet, smoking, urine injections coupled with starvation, stomach amputation) will lead to a healthy body?

If the diet industry's product actually "cured fatness," wouldn't their profits be going down instead of up as more and more people were permanently thin?

Isn't it medically unethical to prescribe something without telling your patients it works less than 5% of the time and the rest of the time has the opposite of the intended effect?

Why do people continue to think shaming people will lead them to health or thinness?

Why do we accept wide variations in things like foot and hand size, nose and lip shape etc. but expect every body to fit into a very narrow proportion of height and weight?

If weight gain isn't proven to cause diabetes and high blood pressure, why would weight loss be recommended as a cure?

Since weight loss ads have to carry a "results not typical" warning, shouldn't doctors have to give patients a similar warning?

Why do people take the time to come to my blog and make death threats?

Does anyone really succeed at hating themselves healthy? If so, is it worth it?

If we've been prescribing dieting since the 1800s and still can't prove it works, shouldn't we be trying something else?

Why is suggesting that healthy habits are the best chance for a healthy body considered controversial?

I'm sure I've forgotten some but that seems like enough nonsense for now. Obviously some of these are oversimplified, but so is the relationship of health and weight in current culture and medical practice. Sometimes things aren't simple. At some point it's time to say that what we've been trying is giving us the exact opposite result, so we need to stop doing it and look for other options.

In the end, I wrote this book because I wish someone had written it for me.

So, what's my deal? I am a professional dancer, choreographer, speaker, blogger, and trained researcher.

I didn't set out to be an Activist. I started out trying to be a fat dancer and choreographer and it turned out I had to be an activist to get it done. That led to my blog. www.danceswithfat.org, which led to more writing and speaking. The activism work I do, including this book, is all meant to accomplish at least one of three things:

Provide access to information about health and debunk myths, while respecting people's right to make their own choices.

Let people know about the Health at Every Size® and Size Acceptance Movements. I'm not trying to make a persuasive argument, but I meet people every day who hated their bodies because they just didn't know there was another option. There is another option.

Ask fat people to consider that they deserve, and can demand, to be treated respectfully in the body they have now, even if they want to lose weight.

Remember, because this is important: No matter where you are today, there are options out there that allow you to love yourself, and pursue health and happiness with the body you have now, whether or not you want to change that body.

There are some important things to get out of the way first:

I am not a doctor, lawyer, or cpa and nothing in this book should be construed as professional medical, legal or financial advice.

I believe people who read my work can think for themselves, and I celebrate their right to do so. It's highly unlikely anyone will agree with every single thing I say in this book. Feel free to take what you like and ignore the rest.

Loving fat people does not mean hating thin ones. I doubt the road to happiness and self-esteem is paved with hypocrisy, so it's no better for me to call someone "skeletal" and say she needs to "eat a sandwich" than it is for someone to say I'm a

fatty who needs to stop eating sandwiches. I'm about respect for
all bodies.

I'm not for or against dieting, weight loss surgery, plastic
surgery, or anything else for anyone else. I am the boss of my
underpants and you are the boss of yours. Therefore I get to
make decisions for my body and you get to make decisions for
yours.

I am for people having access to complete information in order
to make a decision and I feel that since the diet industry makes
so much money selling us their products, they might not be
interested in giving us complete information. It's my goal to
offer some other perspectives you might not hear over the diet
ad din.

I also want to address my Good Fatty/Bad Fatty Conundrum.
This issue only exists because in this culture we are trying to
solve social stigma through weight loss. The cure for social
stigma is ending social stigma; it's not telling the stigmatized
group they should stop making other people want to stigmatize
them. But that hasn't stopped this culture from trying to say
exactly that to fat people.

When I say "Good Fatty," I mean a fat person who is viewed (by
the faction of our society who have decided they are the Judgey
McJudgersons of health) as taking "appropriate steps" to lose
weight or, at the very least, publicly "struggling" with their
weight, thereby earning a modicum of very contingent respect
from someone who would otherwise be a fat hater. It's important
to note that The Good Fatty title is not a self-identity, but rather
a conferred title indicating the fat person is behaving as the fat
hater thinks they should.

If you read my blog regularly, you know I respect other people's decisions about their bodies and health just as I require respect for my decisions. This is not about bashing people who have chosen weight loss. The following anonymous comment was left on a blog I wrote about a series of ugly comments, including death threats, that I had received the previous day:

"…we are not really "fat hating", in fact, if we see someone who asks for help how to lose weight etc we will cheer them on etc and help…"

This is classic Good Fatty language. What this person is really saying is: You deserve the abuse and bullying you are receiving because you won't do what I think you should. You are a Bad Fatty. If you just behave in ways that make me happy, then I will declare you a Good Fatty and I will stop abusing you. However, if you tell me you eat healthy and exercise but you don't achieve the body size I expect, I'll call you a liar to your face and turn the abuse faucet right back on.

This is where my Good Fatty conundrum comes in:

After countless hours of research I believe health is not the same as weight. Health is multi-dimensional. There are some aspects of health within our control and some aspects outside of our control. I believe if I want better health, focusing on healthy habits rather than the size of my body is a completely legitimate, and in fact the best, option.

One of the conundrums I deal with is that I also write about the life I choose as an athlete/dancer. I try to be clear that my lifestyle is driven by my dancing, which means I workout far more than is necessary for just maintaining health. I think sometimes people get confused and think I'm trying to prove I'm a Good Fatty, or I'm trying to say I think people should choose the same thing that I do, or I think I'm better than people who make different choices. That's definitely not what I'm about.

The truth is I don't write for people who want to tell me they think I'm a liar, or I can't possibly be healthy, or I'm a Bad Fatty. I don't write to try to convince anyone of anything. I write what I think is true and I hope that I reach people who have been let down by the weight loss industry. I write for people who get stigmatized by a society that confuses weight and health and has turned fat people into everything from metaphors to scapegoats. I write for people who want to hear a different voice, new ideas, or be supported in making their own choices about their own bodies.

People may try to label us Good Fatties, Bad Fatties, or whatever they want. They may try to convince us that we must gain their approval in order to avoid their abuse. But I think we always have the option to decide we aren't Tinkerbell, and we don't need anyone's applause to live. Then we can opt out of the labeling system for ourselves and each other and demand (and give) basic human respect that is not contingent on anyone's weight or the choices they make for their bodies and their health, even if they aren't doing what we would choose to do or think is best.

How It Starts

It starts with a guess: "You're fat; so I guess you just don't take care of your body."

Add an assumption: "I'll bet you eat tons of junk food and don't exercise."

Make a judgment: "So I think you are lazy and don't care about your body."

Confuse your experience with everyone's experience: "I once gained 10 pounds after a bad breakup I was able to lose it by drinking two chocolate shakes for breakfast and lunch and eating a tiny dinner."

Draw an illogical conclusion: "Since I lost 10 pounds on my first ever diet, you can lose 200 pounds on your 20th diet by doing what I did, just for a longer period of time."

Confuse correlation and causation: "Besides, if you don't lose weight, you'll get diabetes."

Repeat something you've heard a lot but never taken the time to verify: "Plus you cost the workplace billions of dollars–think of the tax dollars!"

Misinterpret the concept of personal responsibility: "You are personally responsible for looking how I want you to look and doing what I want you to do or there should be consequences!"

Make a broad sweeping generalization: "Health at Every Size? It's just like a fatty to eat Twinkies all day and call it healthy!"

Tell other people what they need to do with their bodies: "I don't know how much you're eating or how much exercise you're doing and I don't care about the facts –you need to eat less and exercise more."

By a bit of a hypocrite: "It doesn't matter that I partake in all the behaviors that I criticize in fat people. I'm at a healthy weight so as long as I'm thin I can do whatever I want."

Ignore the facts: "What do you mean there are unhealthy thin people and healthy fat people? I don't want to hear about medical studies and science – you're just justifying your fatness."

Become frustrated and insult us: "Shut up, you're just a big fat fatty."

Repeat this conversation so often that people start to believe it.

I see this exact line of "logic" spun out all the time and once you really look at it , you realize it's a house of cards built on a foundation of toothpicks.

First, if someone's argument starts with a guess then it doesn't really matter what they say afterwards. They absolutely cannot look at someone's body and glean any information other than the size of that body and what their prejudices and preconceived notions about a body that size are.

Second, unless they are also going to start a campaign against Iron Man Triathletes, climbing Everest, sedentary thin people, being a cast member on Jackass, and jaywalkers (since none of these activities prioritize health), they don't get to pick on fat people. Of course, none of it is actually their business at all. Policing other people's bodies is a slippery slope indeed.

Most of these misconceptions could be avoided if people were self-aware enough to honestly answer the questions: "Do I actually know what I'm talking about or am I repeating things that I've never verified for myself?" and "Would I want to be treated the way I'm treating this group of people?" But most people are not this introspective. As a fat person this isn't my fault, but it becomes my problem. What helps me is to remind myself how utterly ridiculous this whole thing is and how much of it is based on guessing, assuming, misinterpreting, repeating without verifying, and just being an ass.

Fortunately, there is a revolution happening, and it's one without guns or knives and very few epic battles. It's a revolution of tiny acts. In the culture we live in, every act of liking ourselves is revolutionary. Get out of bed and don't hate yourself? You are a revolutionary. Go on a walk and enjoy moving your body (despite the possibility of having to deal with idiots?) You are a revolutionary. Enjoyed your lunch without guilt? Viva la revolution! Rest assured, all these acts are adding up. More of us every day are seeing choosing to step away from the self-hate, and soon all of the assuming, misinterpreting, myth repeating people in the world won't be able to stop us. It's an uprising of fatties and our friends. Join in!

My Other Favorite F Word

Pleasantly plump, BBW, more cushion for the pushin', fluffy, big boned, rubenesque, zaftig, person of size. What we call ourselves can be really important.

You may have noticed I am fond of using the word "fat." There are several reasons behind this but predominantly I use it because it was a word used by bullies of every stripe to try to make me feel bad about myself. My use of the word fat as a self-descriptor is my way of telling those bullies they cannot have my lunch money any more.

It's also a way of challenging assumptions. When I'm setting up a business meeting with someone in a coffee shop I tell them to look for the "short, fat, brunette with her hair up in a bun," and they will often say "Oh, don't call yourself fat." Not once has someone said, "Oh, don't call yourself brunette."

I'm fat - I have a lot of adipose tissues. I'm 5'4" and weigh 284 pounds. I'm okay with people calling me fat because they can see I have a lot of adipose tissue, just as I am okay with people calling me a brunette because they can see I have brown hair.

The problem occurs when a whole bunch of judgments and negative connotations come along for the ride. In our culture, fat has become shorthand for any number of negative descriptors: unhealthy, lazy, unattractive, unfit, un-athletic. People dread the idea of appearing fat and go through an incredible amount of discomfort (from being wrapped in plastic wrap and heated, to being encased in so many restrictive undergarments they feel like a sausage and can barely breathe) in an effort to appear smaller or differently shaped...even to look just a *little less* fat.

They sell swimsuits in my size that say "Look 10 pounds slimmer!" Really? What could I possibly be trying to accomplish by looking 274lbs instead of 284lbs?

Of course people have every right to do whatever they want with their bodies and I have absolutely no issue with those choices. I'm just suggesting we examine a culture in which not "looking fat" can reasonably be considered a higher priority than breathing.

I do ask that people think before they talk about bodies negatively. When I hear someone say, "Real women have curves" or "Sticks aren't sexy," I cringe, because I know women who aren't curvy, and that doesn't make them un-real. The very thin women I know don't like to be called names and told they aren't attractive any more than my fat friends and I do.

When I'm trying to be more formal in describing someone else (especially if I don't know their descriptor of choice), I typically go with "person of size," I think it has a lovely ring to it, and it reminds me of "person of distinction," which makes me happy.

If some words still make you want to punch someone in the face, I would suggest you consider trying to take some of the sting away. You can't control what other people call you, but you can control your reactions and how much power those words have over you. One of my blog readers wrote in to say that a particularly unpleasant client, who knew her name just fine, asked for her as "the fat one in the office." She asked me what she should do. If it were me I would have picked up the phone and cheerfully said, "This is the fat one; how can I help you?" without a trace of anger or irony. To me it's the equivalent of saying "Oh, my lunch money? Nope, you can't have that. Sit down and shut up." One could also say, "I understand you asked for me as 'the fat one.' That's completely fine, except we have employees of all sizes here, so to make sure you get the right person you can always ask for me by my name."

In the end, we each get to choose our own descriptors and why we use them, and how much power other people's descriptors have over us.

Myths, Misconceptions and Mixed Messages

The "War on Obesity" has spawned a ton of myths, misconceptions and mixed messages that fat people have to live with every day. They say sunshine is the best disinfectant, so let's shine some light.

Our Big Fat Authority Problem

When I break the cardinal rule of being fat on the internet and read the comments, I'm always shocked at the authority with which complete strangers tell me things about myself that, apparently, I did not know:

You cannot be healthy at [arbitrary weight]

Obesity causes [insert disease never proven to be caused by obesity]

Everyone who is fat will eventually get sick from it

These are three common misconceptions that have been proven false many times over, but I think one of the things that gives them power is that they are stated with authority. Never mind that they are being written by people who get their information from diet commercials and wouldn't know the difference between correlation and causation if it bit them in the ass; we live in a sound bite society, and this type of comment is perfectly suited for that.

The more you learn, the more you know how very few things are certain, and how much is grey rather than black and white. This leads to people like me, who have done our research, saying things like:

"Health is multi-dimensional and includes access, genetics, environment, stress, and behaviors. Weight loss fails 95% of the time in the long term. So for me, I think if I want to be healthy, the best course of action is to practice healthy behaviors rather than trying to change the size and shape of my body."

Then someone else who has not done any research but is relying on "common knowledge" says, "It's impossible to be fat and healthy."

So in the end, I sound like I'm hedging and qualifying and trying to talk around an issue, and they sound direct and authoritative.

This also applies to emotional intelligence. I notice the more emotionally intelligent and mature a person is, the more they realize their experience is not everyone's experience. So I say, "We celebrate X Games athletes who risk their lives every day for a sport. We celebrate people who jump out of helicopters wearing skis, and people who push their bodies to the limit running Iron Man Triathlons. All of those things are physically risky and do not prioritize health. I value health, but that doesn't mean everyone has to make it their first priority, or that people who do the same things I do will have the same results. In the end, I believe in giving people correct information and affordable accessible options, and then respecting their choices as I expect them to respect mine."

And somebody else says, "I lost weight and I'm healthier, so all fat people should lose weight and they'll be healthier too."

Again, I sound like Wordy McWorderson, mayor of Wordsworth, while they appear to be brief and to the point (however erroneous that point might be).

So what is there to do? Rarely do you get points for appearing to complicate an argument. But the situation isn't black and white and I don't want to act like it is. So I've tried to find statements that are short, factual, and that I can say with equal authority, such as:

- You can't look at a person and tell how healthy they are
- There are healthy and unhealthy people of every size
- People of all sizes deserve to be treated with respect

Everybody Knows

The most unscientific phrase in history might be, "Everybody knows…"

We just talked about how to deal with that attitude intellectually, but how do we emotionally deal with constantly being assaulted by sweeping generalizations stated as if they are facts, especially when we know they are wrong. I think people end up repeating these myths and misconceptions for all kinds of reasons including:

- They honestly (but mistakenly) believe what they are saying is proven fact
- It makes them feel better about themselves to speak in absolutes as if they know for sure what is true for everyone
- They lack the intellectual humility to be aware that they could be wrong
- They know they could be wrong but they lack the emotional intelligence to admit it

In any event, dealing with the constant barrage of this can be anything from frustrating to maddening.

These situations often make me think of Galileo. At the core, he was a guy who was looking at the research and saying, "I know everyone believes the sun revolves around the Earth, but I'm looking at the evidence and it does not support that conclusion." So of course the establishment said: "Wow, thank you for bringing this up! We need to look into this—'Hey, everybody, we might be wrong'!"

Wait…no, that's not what happened at all. They made him recant and put him under house arrest for life.

Obviously that put a damper on his social life but it didn't make him any less correct – the Earth does in fact move around the sun and not the other way around.

Galileo is a reminder to me that a majority of people (including those in power) believing something and repeating it endlessly does not indicate that it's true. I like to think I'm part of that tradition – I'm just a woman looking at the evidence and saying I know everyone believes you have to be thin to be healthy, and that everyone who tries hard enough loses weight, but the evidence just doesn't support it.

Instead of parroting what "everybody knows," let's take a look at what nobody knows:

- Nobody can prove that fat actually causes the health issues it gets blamed for; all we know for sure is that they sometimes happen at the same time
- Nobody who says that fat is unhealthy can explain the 51% of overweight adults and 30% of obese adults who are metabolically healthy
- Nobody knows for sure why fat women who aren't concerned about their weight have less physical and

mental illness than those who are – regardless of their weight

- Nobody knows for sure why all of the health problems correlated with being fat are also correlated with being under constant stress
- Nobody can prove why we're getting fatter (and there's actually a lot of argument as to whether or not we are.)
- Nobody knows how healthy fat people would be if they didn't live in a society that constantly stigmatizes you and tells us that we can't possibly be healthy

That's a lot of "nobody knows." So the way I deal with the constant barrage of BS is by reminding myself that people can say, "Everybody knows you just eat less and exercise more and you'll lose weight," or "Everybody knows we're fatter because of fast food/sedentary lifestyle/hormones in food/alien invasion," or "Everybody knows we would all be thin if we would just give up carbs/give up sugar/go vegetarian/go vegan/go paleo/drink most of our meals/swallow a tape worm." But the evidence does not support their hypotheses and so the truth is that what "everybody" knows is--nothing.

We all have opinions and we are entitled to base our choices on our opinions, but that's where it ends. Nobody has the right to tell me personal responsibility means I am personally responsible for making **my** choices based on **their** opinions, and I don't have to prove anything to anyone. So whenever I see one of these comments I picture them dressed up in 17th Century garb writing with a quill, "The sun revolves around the Earth" It puts it right back in perspective for me.

The VFHT

Doctors do it. So do well meaning neighbors, relatives and people on the street. The diet industry does it for profit.

The VFHT: The Vague Future Health Threat.

It sounds like this: "Well, you may be fat and healthy now, but it will catch up to you someday." This is often followed by a triumphant look because this is indefensible, as it's hard to argue with someone who is essentially telling you they are psychic.

The VFHT takes advantage of the fact that everyone is going to die, and tries to convince us that when fat people die it will be because of our fat. I find this to be paternalistic, ignorant, unsupported, and annoying for the following reasons:

1. Typically the person VFHTing me has already inaccurately assessed my current health (i.e., "Nobody can be healthy at your weight") and now they want me to believe they can accurately predict my future health.

2. What is this "it" that will catch up to me? I am not outrunning my fat – it's all right here. I am not a thin woman covered in fat; I am a fat woman who is also a very fit athlete. So what's going to catch up with me: My good blood pressure, cholesterol, glucose and triglycerides? My working out and eating healthy? My strength, stamina, and flexibility?

3. Everyone is going to die. There is a 100% chance. I just happen to live in a culture where it doesn't matter why I die-- someone will blame it on my fat. That doesn't make it true.

4. What if I changed the rules of the lottery so that if you lost, you had to pay the lottery money as a penalty? Now not only is your chance of winning infinitesimally small, but there is a nearly 100% chance you'll end up with LESS money than you had before you bought the ticket. Would you play? Now imagine this isn't your money we're talking about – it's your long term health. There is not a single study that proves any

weight loss method is effective long term, but many studies indicate weight cycling (yo-yo dieting) is less healthy than being obese. Since diets have such an abysmal failure rate, if I go on just two diets where I lose weight and gain it back (and I have an extremely high chance of doing just that both times), I've likely damaged my current good health and endangered my future health on a roll of the dice that was obviously a losing bet from the beginning. The person VFHTing me is asking that I do something they can't prove is possible, for a reason they can't prove is valid, with a very high percentage I'll end up less healthy at the end. I'll pass.

So what do you say to the VFHT?

Here are some possible responses broken down by category.

Quick and simple:

- I find it inappropriate for you to make guesses about my future health.
- My health is not your business. (If, at this point, they bring up tax payer dollars or health care costs, I ask them for an itemized list of things for which their local, state, and federal taxes pay, or health problems people develop for which causation cannot be proven; broken down into categories of things they are happy to pay for, and things they don't want to pay for. If they don't happen to have that list on hand, I let them know I'll be happy to discuss it once they do.)

More detailed/scientific

- I don't know of a single scientific study that shows significant weight loss is possible for the majority of people. So, either cite your research or I'm going to assume I know more about this than you do and you are just talking without actually knowing what you're talking about. (Or "talking out of your ass" depending on my mood.)

- You have no way to know that. Cite your research or I will assume you are putting my health at risk by making recommendations about which you have no actual knowledge or qualifications, which is completely unacceptable to me.

The pointed response (feel free to mix and match questions/responses with boundary statements)

- How dare you make assumptions about my health? You may not discuss my health with me.
- I find you completely unqualified to make that statement. Please keep your opinions about my health to yourself.
- My health is not your business and you are not allowed to comment on it.
- You will immediately stop making guesses and assumptions about my future health or this conversation is over.

Finally, the snarky responses (I don't actually recommend these because I prefer some kind of productive conversation if possible, but it's fun to think about)

- I had no idea you could predict the future! Would you mind giving me tomorrow's lottery numbers?
- Actually the fat doesn't have to catch up with me – I keep it right here…unless you saw some back there that I lost?
- I totally forgot that being thin will make me immortal – thank god you told me or I might have died some day!

- I've been meaning to tell you that I'm actually worried about you. I read on a website that we are about to experience another ice age and without fat stores to keep you alive and warm, you're absolutely going to freeze to death.

Remember you get to choose how people treat you. If you decide they don't get to VFHT you, then you just need to put that plan into action, set boundaries and consequences and get after it.

But You Won't Live the Longest Possible Life

Fat people often hear that we should try to lose weight so we can live a longer, healthier life. I'm not capitulating, in fact I think it's crap, but for the sake of argument let's say it's true.

First, remember there are plenty of people who put themselves in a position to have shorter, less healthy lives:

There are the daring: People who choose to be professional bull riders, race car drivers and stunt people. People who skydive, bungee jump, and white-water raft. People who live fast and die young with a sex, drugs, and rock- and- roll lifestyle. People who try to climb Everest and swim the English Channel.

And we think that's great. In fact, most of the people who engage in the activities above are celebrated. Not because their life will be as long as possible, but because we perceive it will be as full as possible.

There are the otherwise prioritized: Some attorneys, CEOs, social workers, parents and others who are stressed, sleepless, and not eating as well as they should.

We think that's okay because they are driven and dedicated.

There are the lifestylers: People who eat a steady diet of junk food and never workout because it's not important to them.

As long as they stay thin, we are either fascinated by, or oblivious to, this situation.

Then we have one last category. Fat people. Some of us are daredevils, some are otherwise prioritized, some are lifestylers. Many live very healthy lifestyles.

Regardless, people tell us we have to "do something" so we can live a longer, healthier life.

Even if we assume being fat is a choice for every single fat person (and I don't think it is), the treatment is still unequal when compared to others who choose a "risky lifestyle." Nobody is launching a "war against sedentary thin people who only eat fast food." There is no "war on people who don't look both ways before crossing the street." If an NFL linebacker needs two seats on a plane people ask for his autograph. If his fat accountant needs two seats on a plane people ask for her head on a platter.

I lived a diet lifestyle for many years and I know what that looks like for me. Restricting food, working out far beyond what was healthy for my body, losing weight, gaining it back, never being happy with my body or my situation. Dieting failure was my experience and it's what the evidence says is most people's experience.

I think the thing we sometimes forget about is living the happiest life. I chose Health at Every Size for the same reasons I hear people choose to skydive: I think the odds are in my favor, and if not, I know I am choosing the fullest, happiest life – not the longest one. If a healthy diet and exercise aren't enough to keep me healthy then I've made my peace with that because I'm happy, I feel great, and I love my life. I'd rather have fewer years of that than more years of hating my body and beating my head against a strategy that fails 95% of the time and does not guarantee I will live any longer.

I think the odds are in my favor that healthy behavior gives me the best chance at health. And I get to make that choice, just like others get to choose to eat a raw food diet, eat a low carb diet, or whatever they want. And maybe I'll die of a heart attack at 40 and wonder if dieting would have given me more time. Or maybe one of these people will get hit by a bus at 40 and wonder what cake tastes like. Or maybe we can hang out when we're 90 and talk about how both of our health choices were valid. Either way, we'll be living with the consequences of our own choices and that's exactly as it should be.

But But But Syndrome

I am always a little shocked when people's assumptions about fat people are directly contradicted with evidence, and then rather than question their own assumptions they try to discount or completely ignore the evidence. I call this "But But But syndrome." For example:

Kelly Gneiting is a 400 pound trained sumo wrestler who completed a marathon. The responses to this achievement on internet running forums included, "At 405 lbs he probably has a very difficult time just walking." Yeah - obviously not that difficult since he just completed a marathon in a respectable time. But I don't think this commenter even thought it through because they are too busy trying not to challenge their assumptions. What they are really saying is, "But but but I like to think of fat people as lazy and un-athletic, and I want to keep it that way - by sheer idiocy if necessary."

Talented Yoga teacher Anna Guest-Jelley wrote a beautiful letter about yoga and Health at Every Size. The responses on Internet yoga websites included, "Too many people practicing now are overweight and not fit. Justifying obesity is a disorder." Which, when translated through the But But But-ometer actually says: "But but but I like to feel superior and think being thin gives me the right to dictate who is a "real" yogini; therefore I will say that any other way of thinking constitutes a disorder."

This happens on my blog when I talk about being a healthy athlete and people call me a liar. "But but but I don't want to be wrong so I'll just say I'm a better witness to your experience than you are."

Even doctors do it. Many fat people I know, including me, have had doctors try to prescribe blood pressure and cholesterol medicine BEFORE testing our blood pressure or cholesterol. And upon finding out they are normal they turn to the VFHT. "But but but I don't want to look like an idiot so even though my laziness and lack of knowledge led to me prescribing medicine that would have harmed you physically, I'm going to try to convince you that even though I'm harmfully wrong today I'll be right eventually."

It's not just fit fat people who are VFHT'd, and this isn't a recent thing. Again, when Galileo looked at the research and agreed with Copernicus that the Earth revolved around the sun, he was sentenced to "formal imprisonment at the pleasure of the Inquisition" which was commuted to house arrest for the rest of his life. Publishing of his current or future works was forbidden. "But but but we don't want to be wrong, so shut that guy up!"

In my experience, when you openly practice Behavior Centered Health, even if you very specifically avoid trying to impress your views on anyone else, it challenges people's assumptions and stereotypes in a way that makes them uncomfortable. So you have to be aware of But But But Syndrome, because some of those people are going to do everything they can to hold on to their assumptions and stereotypes, even if it means attacking you.

For the record, I think the best cure for "But But But Syndrome" is for these people to Butt Butt Butt Out.

Looking at Someone's Size is Not a Diagnosis

Who can resist a sentence that starts "The dictionary defines..."? I hope you can't because...

The dictionary defines diagnosis as "the act or process of identifying or determining the nature and cause of a disease or injury through evaluation of patient history, examination, and review of laboratory data."

Notice it doesn't say: "The act of looking at someone fully clothed, making guesses about their health, and medicating, shaming and/or stigmatizing them based on your conclusions."

That's because that would be stupid. Except it's exactly what modern diagnostic techniques are doing. They're taking a ratio of weight and height and making guesses about people's health, eating habits, physical fitness, etc.

Maybe those techniques could be justified in 1832, but considering the actual diagnostic tools available to us now, looking at someone's body and making guesses is not only behind the times, it's completely unnecessary. This doesn't just hurt fat people either. Obviously if doctors gave every obese person medication for Type 2 Diabetes, it would be a massive over-reaction, since we know many obese people don't have Type 2 Diabetes and therefore we know obesity is not an automatic affirmative diagnosis for the disease. What the medical profession often forgets, in their hurry to assign medical conditions to fat people, is the tremendous disservice they are doing to all the thin people who have Type 2 Diabetes but have their symptoms ignored, or aren't being tested for the disease, just because their doctor thinks a thin body constitutes an automatic negative diagnosis.

The thing about body size is that it's never an affirmative or negative diagnosis of anything. There may be some things more strongly correlated to certain sizes of bodies, but that doesn't mean those things are always present in a body that size. The only thing you can tell from the size of someone's body is how big they are and what your preconceived notions about their size are. Trying to diagnose anything else is a shamefully lazy way to practice health care.

If someone is saying a thin woman must have anorexia and needs to eat a sandwich, or a fat woman must have diabetes and should put down the sandwich, they should check their assumptions. There are too many healthy and unhealthy people of every shape and size for these kinds of assumptions to hold up. And while we're talking about it, why are other people concerning themselves with our health – it's none of their business?

Confusing body size with actual health issues is dumb and dangerous no matter who is making the mistake.

The Truth about "Diabesity"

The term Diabesity® was coined and copyrighted by a group called "Shape Up America" which, according to its website is "a high profile national initiative to promote healthy weight and increased physical activity in America… [i]nvolving a broad-based coalition of industry, medical/health, nutrition, physical fitness, and related organizations and experts."

But if you look more deeply you'll find they received millions of dollars of sponsorship money from corporations including Weight Watchers International, Jenny Craig and Slim*Fast. In fact, Slim*Fast paid for a one-page free-standing insert in Sunday newspapers that featured Shape Up America on one side and an ad for Ultra Slim*Fast (that included the Shape Up America logo) on the other. They have also accepted at least $100,000 from Wyeth-Ayerst, a pharmaceutical company that makes a number of diet drugs.

So while I applaud the portmanteau, I have to come down against the intentional confusion of weight and health for profit.

This became a big deal because news outlets starting reporting the "diabesity epidemic" and then everybody thought they could tell from someone's weight whether or not they have type 2 diabetes, which is simply not true.

Being overweight doesn't mean you'll get diabetes. One of the ways I know is because the American Diabetes Association says on their website:

"Myth: If you are overweight or obese, you will eventually develop type 2 diabetes.

Fact: Being overweight is a risk factor for developing this disease, but other risk factors such as family history, ethnicity and age also play a role. Unfortunately, too many people disregard the other risk factors for diabetes and think weight is the only risk factor for type 2 diabetes. Most overweight people never develop type 2 diabetes, and many people with type 2 diabetes are at a normal weight or only moderately overweight. "

Fatness is not a disease. It's not a diagnosis. Obesity as we currently define it is simply a ratio of weight and height. By this definition almost the entire NFL is headed toward diabetes. Fatness is a body size; it is not a behavior or set of behaviors. There are fat people who exercise and those who don't. There are fat meat eaters, fat vegetarians and fat vegans. There are healthy fat people and unhealthy thin people.

Type 2 Diabetes is not a body size. It is a disease. It's a disease that happens in people of all sizes, it is very manageable with proper treatment. Proper treatment includes food choices, exercise, and medication and does not require weight loss.

Yet instead of prescribing the same evidence-based behavior-centered treatment and medication that they give to thin people, when it comes to fat people doctors just prescribe weight loss. When people fail at weight loss, as we should expect they will based on the data, doctors blame them and tell them to try again. What if Viagra only worked 5% of the time and doctors kept prescribing it and then blamed the other 95% of the guys for not trying hard enough? In medicine, if a prescription doesn't work 95% of the time, they work to develop a new solution; they don't blame the patient and tell them to keep taking the prescription but try harder.

Then there's the issue of testing bias. An organization funded by people who profit from weight loss has made the idea of diabesity so pervasive that doctors test their fat patients for Type 2 diabetes even if they have no symptoms, but often wait until long after symptoms occur to test their thin patients. If population A is tested for a disease and population B is not, nobody should be surprised that we find more incidences of the disease in population A.

I'm a fan of health. Why can't we be for health? Why do we have to create a culture of guilt, shame and blame? Why not be honest: Even if weight loss would solve these health problems (and we don't know if it would), we don't know how to actually achieve it so it's time to go looking for another solution.

If we let go of the notion that weight loss works, we would pull our health out of the wallets of the diet industry (including the diet industry disguised as non-profit organizations like Shape Up America). Once we do that, we'll find ourselves with billions of dollars to create access to affordable, healthy foods; movement options we enjoy; and affordable evidence-based healthcare. Imagine what kind of health we could have as a nation if we actually focused on health!

Their Money and Our Fat Asses

"As long as my insurance and tax dollars continue to pay for there [sic] diabetes, and heart disease, I'll continue to feel justified in telling every overweight person I see that they need to lose weight. Shame is powerful and their fat is costing me real money"

This argument, straight from a comment on my blog, is another thing based on the assumption that all fat people are unhealthy and are going to get diabetes and/or heart disease. Let's look at this two ways. First by looking at the reality/truth, and then by presuming these assumptions are true:

Reality:

I know I'm repeating myself and I think it bears repeating - nobody can tell how healthy a person is by looking at them. There is simply no such thing as a healthy weight. There are healthy fat people and unhealthy thin people. There are physically active fat people and sedentary thin people. There are fat people who eat a well balanced diet and thin people who eat like crap. Almost everyone has a thin friend who eats a ton of crappy food and stays thin, and typically people accept that. But let a person eat well and still be fat and, in my experience, those same people will call them a liar. People seem to think our fat bodies show our "sins" and they seem to think that gives them the right to judge us or make assumptions about how many tax dollars we cost. This goes right back to people being too lazy to look at actual health, and people being way over-interested in body size while not being nearly as concerned about people who don't look both ways before crossing the street or who don't get enough sleep. My fat body is not a symbol of anything, and it's certainly not proof of a tax burden, which is why this argument falls apart minutes after it is made.

But let's pretend the assumption is true.

In that case: I'm fat, so I'm unhealthy. But…

I've never even smoked a cigarette. And yet my tax dollars go to all the people who get health problems related to smoking.

I don't drink. I've never even been drunk. And yet my tax dollars pay for cirrhosis, drunk driving accidents and alcohol poising.

I've never done drugs. And yet my tax dollars pay for people whose lives and bodies fall apart due to drug abuse.

I look both ways before I cross the street. And yet I have to pay for people who get run over after failing to do so.

I exercise regularly – cardio, flexibility, and resistance training. Yet my tax dollars will pay for people (of all shapes and sizes) whose sedentary lifestyle leads to health problems.

Marathoners drop dead of heart attacks. People who do everything "right" die of diseases to which they were genetically predisposed. Shit happens and our tax dollars pay for it and that's just how it goes.

Bottom line:

…even if they could prove being fat makes us unhealthy (which they can't);

…even if they had a method that was scientifically proven to lead to successful long term weight loss (which they don't);

… even if there was proof that losing weight would make us healthier (which there isn't);

and…

… even if they were going to go around yelling at smokers, drinkers, jay walkers, and thin people who don't exercise (which they aren't) this slope is still too slippery.

And that doesn't take into account the reality that their premise is completely flawed, their assumptions are faulty, and their method of shaming people is utterly ineffective, since you can't make someone hate themselves healthy.

So I think it would be dandy if they would just shut up.

Mixed Messages

Fat people today live in a culture that gives us an unbelievable number of mixed messages. Some are nuanced and some are obvious, but they are all correctable. Let's look at some.

Your body makes you unattractive and unhealthy. You should be ashamed of the reflection you see. Now, go take good care of your body!

I think this one is the most prevalent. People don't take care of things they hate, whether it's a gift from their mother-in-law or their body. People don't care for something they don't think is worthy of care. So these people who are trying to hate us healthy can shut up already! Every body is beautiful and amazing, and if you disagree, please feel free to apply your beliefs to your own body and leave the rest of us alone.

We are fighting a war against you. Say thank you; it's for your own good!

Around my blog we call this "Pulling a Jillian" (after Jillian Michaels, the trainer on The Biggest Loser who prides herself on physically, verbally and emotionally bullying her clients "for their own good"). Abuse is never, ever, called for. Wars have casualties and if you are fighting the war against obesity then you'd better be ready to accept responsibility for the injuries (mental and physical), deaths, and collateral damage you leave in your wake. Or you could fight for healthy options, make choices for yourself, and respect the choices of others – a much more casualty-free way of being.

When you go to the doctor they will humiliate you and provide subpar treatment. Now stop being such a drain on the healthcare system.

According to research from Yale, over 50% of doctors find their fat patients "awkward, weak-willed and unlikely to comply with treatment". This leads to fat people getting less time with the doctor and less respect. Often doctors will ignore whatever we came in for, do absolutely no diagnostic work, diagnose us as fat without so much as touching us, give us a treatment protocol of weight loss, and send us on our way. I'm not too worried about being a drain on a healthcare system that treats me like yesterday's bedpans.

If you don't work out, we will complain that you are sedentary. If you do work out, we will make fun of you for how you look working out. Now, go out there and exercise because it's good for your health!

Why is it always the same people who assume (out loud) that I don't exercise who also have a problem with how I look when I exercise? I would prefer they just leave me alone…but at minimum they should probably choose one or the other.

Happy Fat People are NOT like a V8 Commercial

You've probably seen it before. A fat person has the audacity to do something awesome and get publicity for it and immediately someone brings up the concern that they are "promoting obesity." I've observed this happen almost any time a fat person is shown in the media being good at anything or having any kind of success not tied to weight loss. It is also among the most ridiculous things I've ever heard. As if someone will see me dancing and think "I wish I could dance like that. The secret must be her obesity. Screw dance lessons; I'm going to try to get fat!" That's insulting to my years of hard work and training, and it's insulting to your intelligence. As if it's the new V8 commercial: millions of thin people will see one of us being successful in some way, smack their foreheads and say "I could've been fat!"

Promoting a body size is what got us into this mess in the first place. I think being thin might be the most aggressively promoted idea of my lifetime, and while it hasn't made everyone thin (in fact, if you believe the statistics, the majority of people are not thin), it has insidiously created a second class of citizens. The completely wrong idea that the only path to health dead ends at a thin body has led to fat people being criticized for being unhealthy, lazy, unattractive, mass Twinkie eaters. And as soon as someone shows a fat person who doesn't fit the stereotype they get shouted down by the ridiculous notion that they're "promoting obesity".

And if you are a fat person who doesn't fit the stereotype, I have noticed that often, rather than logically thinking, "Wow, I should really check my own stereotypes about fat people," people will simply ignore all the evidence and simply state loudly that you DO fit the stereotype. I can't believe people can watch me dance, hear me repeatedly say that my Health at Every Size practice is about eating healthy and exercising, and still say I am promoting an unhealthy lifestyle. What is the hell is wrong with these people? Mary Lou Retton is a famous speaker and nobody accused her of promoting shortness.

Look, if someone sees a fat person and immediately thinks all they do is sit around and eat Twinkies, then THEY have a problem: they are a bigot who stereotypes fat people. If the sight of a fat person being athletic makes them angry, then they have some very serious issues to deal with. If they think happy successful fat people are promoting obesity, then they are dangerously delusional. Happy successful fat people are not promoting obesity; they are promoting being happy and successful.

If we follow the logic that putting fat people in the public eye as anything other than a stereotype or an ad for stomach amputation is "promoting obesity," what they are really saying is fat people should never get to see anyone who looks like us in a positive light. To think this way is to seriously believe the best thing they can do for fat people is make sure we never see people who look like us being active or successful or happy, but rather we should only see ourselves represented as caricatures of negative stereotypes – lazy, unattractive, lonely failures. How messed up is? How cruel? First they tell fat people we are all lazy, unsuccessful, and unlovable, then they purposefully hide all the evidence to the contrary under the guise of not "promoting obesity," then they use that lack of evidence to "prove" all fat people are lazy, unsuccessful and unlovable. Then they make billions of dollars promising to make fat people thin, or keep thin people from getting fat.

We have GOT to stop promoting any body size at all. We need to show, and celebrate, the diversity of the human experience, and that includes all colors, shapes, sizes, sexual orientations, and levels of activity--from athletes to couch potatoes; everybody. Our diversity is what makes us strong – it's what makes us survivors. Pretending otherwise for their own profit ought to buy them a special place in hell.

I'm just happy there are people standing up to this preposterous notion, who are brave and strong enough not to cave in to the pressure, and who are getting fat role models out into the light where they belong. I'm proud and thankful for all the fatties who brave the whole lotta ugly that comes at them from a never-ending parade of stupid to live their lives out loud and be role models for all of us!

Oh The Things People Say

When you are a fat person in a culture that thinks it can look at you and know everything there is to know about your health, eating, exercise habits, and work ability, you are going to hear some crazy stuff. Like the Boy Scouts always say: the best plan is to be prepared, so let's examine some of the most common offenders:

Fat People Need to Have More Personal Responsibility

One of the things I hear a lot is that my body is the result of a "lack of personal responsibility." But I don't think people really mean that I don't take personal responsibility. If they read my blog, they would be aware that I take complete responsibility for my behavior; I just don't buy into the thin=healthy idea. I've done tons of research, drawn conclusions, and created a health strategy I implement in living my life. If that's not personal responsibility, I don't know what is.

I think what people mean to say is that my idea of health doesn't match theirs and they think I am personally responsible for doing what they want me to do to make them happy with who I am and how I look. That doesn't work for me, since it's my health and my body. Let's not forget their plan for me is based entirely on guessing, assuming, and judging.

These people want to look at my body and guess about my choices, make assumptions about my level of "personal responsibility" and decide they have right to judge me and say rude, cruel and accusatory things about my health and its impact on our society. Unfortunately their guesses are erroneous, their assumptions are flawed, and their judgments are inappropriate. People cannot look at us and determine how much personal responsibility we are taking. And even if they could, it's not their business whether someone else is making healthy choices for themselves; that's why it's called personal responsibility.

So what do you say to this?

The long version:

I typically go with "Personal responsibility doesn't mean I'm personally responsible for doing what you want me to do or looking how you want me to look. I'm comfortable with my choices and am not soliciting outside opinions."

The short form:

"I'm going to ask you to mind your own business and I'll mind mine."It's for Your HealthEvery fat person I know has heard this one: "You need to lose weight for your health."

The problem with people who torment us "for our own good" is that, unlike the bully whose conscious will hopefully tell him that it's not ok to beat up kids for money, the "for our own good" bully does it with the blessing of her or her conscious – they are able to justify their inappropriate bullying and meddling as "noble." It is not.

This is known in the blogosphere as "concern trolling." It makes the assumption that as fat people we can't possibly be the best witnesses to our own experiences or make the best choices for ourselves. It's paternalism at its worst, disguised as concern. Even if the accuser had a legitimate concern, do they actually think we've somehow missed the message that thin is healthy? They are allowed to be concerned, but that's their issue to deal with, not ours.

So what do you say?

I keep it simple with this one:

"I appreciate your concern, but I'm very comfortable with my research and choices and I'm not soliciting outside opinions. " I think that sentence clearly and politely conveys that the captain has turned on the sit down and shut up light.

Oops, That's Not a Compliment

Sometimes people, even if they mean well, can really show us the back hand of a compliment.

I was at a meeting wearing a skirt and a sleeveless shirt, which is rare at this meeting because it's typically really cold. The responses I got provide a handy guide by which people who want to compliment us can judge whether or not they are doing it right:

"Look at you, rocking a dress!" (Said positively, no hint of sarcasm.)

Compliment. Well done.

*"***Oh** *(makes pensive face)***, I didn't think you wore dresses. I actually think pants suit you better***."*

Nope, not a compliment. Not a thing to say at all really. Maybe should have used their inner monologue on this one.

"Wow, I don't think I've seen you wear a skirt before. You look so cute."

Compliment. That's how you do it!

"I just wanted to tell you that I think you're very brave to wear a sleeveless shirt, I always feel like my arms are too fat" (said by someone less than half my size).

Swing and a miss, I'm afraid. I appreciate that they've made it clear this is your issue and not mine, but really if their attempt at a compliment starts with "you're so brave" and doesn't end with "for fighting off those wild animals," they should just skip it.

So what do you do when you're on the receiving end of a failed compliment? I'll leave it up to you to decide the ratio of rudeness to cluelessness in the comment, but here is a spectrum of answers:

Simple and clean:

Say "Thank you" like you really didn't get any negative implications and walk away.

Gentle correction:

Thank you; I'm sure you meant that as a compliment and I appreciate it.

Correction and Substitution:

"Brave" isn't really a compliment. I'd take, "You look great," though!

Confrontational:

You know, that really sounded like a back-handed compliment. Was that your intention?

Food Police on Parade

Ah the joys of having people question our food choices! "Do you really need to eat that?" is certainly the one I heard most often from my family. Another, more specific, form of concern trolling, this assumes I hadn't really thought my food choices through and therefore need the help of a dining companion to decide what foods I want and how much of them I should consume.

This question is custom-made to make us feel ashamed. I think it's typically asked for one of about three reasons:

Judgment

The person asking the question has decided it is their job to pass judgment on your activities. Being too cowardly to directly state their opinion, they use this question as a mode of passive aggression to "make you admit it to yourself"

Power/Superiority

Remember some people never got past Junior High and nothing makes them feel as powerful as judging someone else and then making that person feel like crap. Maybe because they are drowning in...

Insecurity

The person asking the question perhaps struggles with their weight and their own guilt about eating, and since they feel guilty for enjoying food, they think you should feel guilty about it, too, or they want to deflect attention from their behavior to yours.

The degree of difficulty in discerning someone's intent in this sort of thing can range from "no duh" to "who the hell knows?" I suggest it doesn't matter why they are asking it; I am not okay with being asked, and I get to choose how I allow people to treat me.

So you're at a holiday meal, you reach for the mashed potatoes and someone asks the dreaded question: "Do you need to eat that?" The table falls silent, waiting for your reply. What do you say?

First, I would suggest you quell your rage and resist the urge to say: "Yes, I do need these mashed potatoes. Did you need to marry that jerk?"

Second, as with most situations in which a person lashes out at you, remember this is about their issues and has nothing to do with you. If emotions well up, consider that you may be feeling embarrassed and/or sorry for them rather than ashamed of your own actions.

Now find your happy (or at least your non-homicidal) place, and try one of these:

Quick and Simple (said with finality):

- Yes (and then eat it)

- No (and then eat it)

Answer with a Question (I find it really effective to ask these without malice, with a tone of pure curiosity. If you're not in the mood to have a dialog, skip these.):

- Why would you think that's your business?
- What made you think I want you to police my food intake?
- I thought you were an accountant; are you also a dietitian?

Pointed Response (be ready with a consequence if the behavior continues):

- I find that inappropriate and offensive
- What I eat is none of your business, and your commenting on it is unacceptable to me
- I have absolutely no interest in discussing my food intake with you
- What do you mean by "need"? Are you asking if my glycogen stores are depleted? If I am near starvation? If my body at this moment requires the precise nutrients delivered by cornbread stuffing covered in gravy? Or do you feel fostering a relationship with food that is based on guilt and shame is in my best interest?

Cathartic (but probably not particularly useful if you want to create an opportunity for honest dialog):

- Yes, because dealing with your rudeness is depleting my glycogen stores at an alarming rate
- If I want to talk to the food police, I'll call 911
- Thanks for trying to give me your insecurities, but I was really hoping to get a Wii this year

- No, but using my fork to eat helps to keep me from stabbing you with it

Do Something About It

"If you want people to stop teasing you because you're fat, do something about it."

"Do something" in this scenario means "lose weight." This is the tip of an iceberg of crap. The idea here is that the solution to shaming, harassing and stigmatizing behavior is for the victim to change themselves and hope it gains them the approval of the person doing the shaming, harassing, and stigmatization, and they will then choose another victim.

So what do you say?

> That's bullshit! (You can leave that part out.) The solution to social stigma is not weight loss, it's ending social stigma. I'm not obligated to look how someone else wants me to look to be treated with respect.

You're Just a Quitter

"This whole Fat Acceptance/Health at Every Size thing is just quitting, because dieting is hard."

One of the most difficult things for me when I decided to stop dieting and pursue Health at Every Size was the idea that I was being a quitter. I have never backed down from anything because it was difficult or the odds were stacked against me.

Whether it was in sports, school, or business, I've spent my life doing things other people told me were impossible.

So when I first found out dieting had only a 5% chance of success, I decided I would beat the odds. I continued to try, but nothing worked. I didn't want to be a quitter; I wanted to believe I could be in the 5% if I just worked hard enough.

I believed people who didn't succeed at diets were just weak-willed. I believed weight was a simple matter of calories in/calories out. I believed if I could create a calorie deficit with a combination of calorie restriction and activity then I would lose weight permanently. So I didn't understand why I kept creating a deficit but didn't lose weight, or couldn't keep it off. I've since learned it just doesn't work that way. The body is much more complex than a calories in/calories out model. The human body, it turns out, is a bit more complicated than a lawnmower.

That led to another realization –this wasn't just about hard work or force of will. This wasn't about starving more or running more sprints. This wasn't about my will; it was about my body. A body I hated because it wouldn't get smaller, instead of appreciating for doing everything I had ever asked of it.

I started to do more and more research, and everything I found turned up the same results: Intentional weight loss fails almost all the time, and there is no proof it will lead to health even if it succeeds. However, weight-cycling (yo-yo dieting) is very hard on the system, and studies show it leads to long-term health problems. Dieting began to look more and more like playing Russian roulette with my good health using a 95% loaded gun.

When I found Health at Every Size, I realized my dieting lifestyle didn't make sense. Since I ran my own businesses, sometimes people will ask me why I gave up on weight loss and not on being an entrepreneur when the odds of success are similar. I started one business that was going great until there was a regulation change that made our business model non-viable, so I shut it down. I didn't feel like a quitter. Plenty of people tried to tell me the business could be saved, but I did the research and made the best decision I could based on facts and logic.

For me, that's exactly what Health at Every Size was and is: An intelligent decision based on information and logic.

What I've learned is that I'm fine gambling when it comes to money and love, but not when it comes to my health. I think feeding my body good, healthy food and doing movement I enjoy is much more likely to make me healthy than trying to make my body smaller.

So what do you say when someone accuses you of being a quitter?

> I'm not quitting so much as I'm opting out of a social construct supported by a $60 Billion a year industry that has an abysmal success rate.

> Call it whatever you want, I've found an option that lets me take care of my body and like it at the same time. I'm comfortable with my choice.

> It makes sense to me that if I want healthy I should focus on healthy habits and not on changing the size and shape of my body.

> Calling me a quitter? Seriously? Next are you going to double dog dare me to diet? Make "bock bock" chicken

noises? I think I'll stick with my logical, rational choices. Thanks anyway for the peer pressure.

Just Too Fat

Someone left a comment on my blog that said: "Being a little overweight is okay, but at some point you're just too fat."

Ok, how can I put this delicately? Who the hell does this person think they are?

Maybe it makes them feel important and superior to run around doling out acceptance to those who they deem worthy, but I remain unimpressed. How exaggerated must their sense of self-importance be to think it should be their job to decide what body size is appropriate for someone else?

I think it's a bad idea to tell other people how they need to live their lives. I think we should probably confine ourselves to saying "This is how I live, it works great for me", and then we can shut up and respect other people's right to make choices, just like we want our choices respected. If they want our advice, I think it's safe to assume we'll be among the very first to know.

So, what can we say to this?

> I don't think it's really your business to tell me what size I should be.

> This seems like a slippery slope – who gets to decide how big anyone else gets to be? Do we really want to become people who police other people's bodies?

> I didn't know you were appointed as a special body judge. Was there a ceremony? Was it nice?

The Bottom Line

At this point in time I'm much less concerned that other people figure out that fat people deserve respect and much more concerned that fat people know they deserve respect. You can't control other people, but you can control your reactions and set your own boundaries. Being prepared ahead of time means a much greater chance you'll leave happy with your reactions, and they'll leave with something to think about.

Fatty Fashion

Does This Chapter Make Me Look Fat?

"Does this [article of clothing] make me look fat?"

I've heard it from friends, relatives, on commercials, sitcoms, and movies.

I've never met anyone who wanted to be on the receiving end of this inquiry.

Allow me to make a case for just striking this question from all of human speech, based on my contention that it has never helped anyone, in any way, ever.

First of all, unless someone is wearing the Harry Potter Invisibility Cloak or is a Predator, they can generally assume they will look fat or not based upon whether or not they are fat. This is information to which they should have been privy prior to getting dressed.

Considering the above, how many times are they going to change their outfit if the answer is a consistent yes? Does it have any relation whatsoever to the time at which they are supposed to arrive at wherever they are dressed to go? Specifically, how "not fat" do they have to look before we can leave for the damn movie?

If getting where we are going on time is more important to me than whether or not that baby doll dress makes your tummy look poochy (it probably does; that's what they do), what are my options?

If I think you look both fat and attractive, will this create some sort of [false] paradox in your brain that will cause it to explode? If a bunch of people think other people look fat and attractive, would it create some sort of Vortex of [False] Paradoxical Doom?

What is the definition of fat? Absent some kind of clarification, the person to whom this question has been addressed is set up to fail from the start. Are they asking if that bubble skirt makes their hips look bigger than they are in real life? (Yes, by design.) Or do they want to know if the clothes make them look like you have a specific body fat percentage or BMI? (If that's the case, then I highly recommend Kate Harding's BMI Project http://kateharding.net/bmi-illustrated/ to show the futility of that exercise.)

That's it, I rest my case.

I humbly suggest that your body is amazing. Just as it is. The way I can tell is that you are alive – your lungs breathing; your heart beating; your eyes blinking and reading or your ears are listening to this. Even if you want to change the size and shape of it, it's still the body you are living in now, 100% of the time. I respectfully submit that spending time asking other people if it looks fat probably won't help with anything.

The Skinny Mirror Fallacy

Our culture encourages us to blame our bodies if clothes don't fit - to consider our size and shape to have "flaws" and "problem areas." But we are told to give the credit to our clothes if we do manage to look good.

We say, "These jeans don't look good on me because my ass is too big."

We say, "These jeans make my ass look good."

Why do we blame our bodies when clothes don't fit well, but turn around and give credit to the clothes when they do?

We bemoan our perceived imperfections in the mirror, and if we, by some miracle, like the way we look, we call it a "skinny mirror."

Our poor bodies don't get any credit at all. What if we thought of our bodies as perfect and anything that doesn't work for us as wrong?

I've watched every episode of the show "The Making of the Dallas Cowboys Cheerleaders." I'm revealing this slightly embarrassing personal detail for a reason. In each season they have an episode where the candidates try on the uniform. It turns out their uniform only fits a very specific body type, so some of the girls (who absolutely conform to the stereotypical American ideal of beauty) hate the way they look and, indeed, are cut from the team because the uniform doesn't "look right" on them. The women are often devastated, and even though the people who are running the camp explain that the uniform only looks good on a very specific body type, the candidates almost always blame themselves.

The politics of cheerleading are the subject for another book. What I'm trying to point out is that this attitude isn't just isolated to people of size. What I'm suggesting for all of us is that we consider the idea that it might not be us at all. If you don't like the way a pair of pants looks, consider it's not you...it's the pants.

If you look fantastic in a pair of pants, then consider that it's you – your awesome rocking body--that is making mere pants look sexy. They sure as hell didn't look that good on the rack!

Consider appreciating your body for all of its awesomeness, and forgiving the things that just aren't good enough for you and your fantastic body.

Tyra Banks Shows Us What Not to Do

I stumbled onto a post by Tyra Banks talking about ways to pose for pictures to hide our "flaws," using her own "flaws" as an example. Nothing like someone who made her living being beautiful telling us that she has flaws to make us feel like we should be wearing a burlap sack while adjusting to life as a shut-in. In this scenario her fixes included ways to:

Make your waist look smaller

Make it look like your thighs don't touch

Make your calves look bigger

Of course we're all familiar with the obsession with small waists and thin thighs, but calves that are too small? I never even knew that was a thing!

I may go my whole life not understanding how parts of our bodies can be considered flawed. In the "before" picture in the article, Tyra's apparently too-small calves seem to be holding her up without incident. Her forehead does a fine job of bridging the gap between her eyebrows and her hair.

I was complaining about this to a friend who said "Well, this is fashion – it's what they have to do."

So let's talk about fashion, then, shall we? First of all, I'm not a fatshionista at all. While I understand the art in it and absolutely appreciate people who are into fashion, it's just not my thing.

That said, I have no problem with clothing going in and out of style but I have a massive problem with our bodies, or parts of them, going in and out of style. You are welcome to do anything to your body that you want, but let's realize that we are buying into this system and allowing it to continue and if we don't like it we can stop anytime we want. A few examples to get us started:

Waif/Athletic/Curvy are not fashion statements. They are body types. See also Ectomorph/Mesomorph/Endomorph. It's effing science! Your body is your body; appreciate it.

Lips are not a fashion statement. Why are people willingly using a product called "Snake Bite," gritting their teeth through the pain while it makes their lips swell? Swelling is not good – it is a sign of INJURY. Maybe it's time to get a grip and an ice pack while considering that your lips are perfect just as they are.

Tanning is bad for you. Bad Bad Bad Bad Bad. Skin bleaching is bad for you. Bad Bad Bad Bad Bad. Your natural skin color is beautiful on you. Do you know how I know that? Because it's your NATURAL skin color.

Botox is botulism. Well, that's not entirely accurate – Botox is a neurotoxin produced by the botulism bacteria (clostridium botulinum) that causes paralysis.

Oh, it's not actually Botulism – it's a neurotoxin that causes paralysis? I feel way better about this; go ahead and inject away!

No, wait…don't. I just remembered it's a **neurotoxin that causes freaking paralysis**. I think I'll just keep the lines on my forehead.

And what is with all of this hair drama? If you like to change your look with color, products, etc., that's awesome - knock yourself out. If you are walking around exhausted because you get up two hours early to straighten your hair since curly hair is "out," maybe it's time to rock your curls.

In the end I think it's all about doing what makes you happy. If your stomach is girdled, your lips are swollen, and your hair is fried, as long as it makes you happy I say go for it. However, I think it might be worth it to give some thought to source of that happiness. Is it that you truly want thicker lips, or is it that you feel like you need to fit into an artificial, arbitrary, standard of beauty? Is that okay? The answer is up to you, of course, but I do think it's worth a thought.

Rejoice, It's Swimsuit Season!

It seems almost every woman I know, of any size, starts to have panic attacks the first time she sees swimsuits out on the floor of her favorite store; their pesky cheerfulness belying their greater purpose of prodding us into going on insane cabbage soup diets and considering a move to Alaska.

Here are some reasons that I rock a swimsuit:

1. Because it's my BODY. I live with it 100% of the time. It does awesome things for me like breathing, walking, and swimming and I decided long ago that I am not going to allow anyone to convince me to hate or be ashamed of something I am with 100% of the time for the rest of my life. I get to choose how I feel about my body, I am the only person who gets to

decide that. Nobody else can make me feel good or bad about my body; it's on me.

2. Because it's a pool, and when you go to the pool, you wear a swimsuit. It's not for vanity – it's practical. Once when I was at the pool in my gym, there was a "thin to average" woman (probably a size 8 or 10) in a large t-shirt with a towel wrapped around her legs all the way to her ankles. She scooted to the edge of the pool and, in a move that I can only describe as ninja-esque, threw the towel behind her as she jumped into the water as fast as she could while grabbing a kickboard off the side.

Her Crouching Tiger Hidden Swimwear moves could not mask the fact that she was wearing control top pantyhose under her suit. She looked at me and said "Nobody should have to see these legs without hose on!" Before I could reply, she realized her shirt was caught on the side railing. Then her pantyhose got caught on her kickboard. While I swam laps she spent most of the time dealing with being in the water with a giant shirt and pantyhose. I am simply not willing to put up with that kind of hassle or have my technique interrupted by a ginormous swatch of cloth - which, when it is wet, hides nothing anyway - and pantyhose, which I will not wear under any circumstances in the world, ever.

3. Because I do not care if people are offended by my body. People are allowed to be offended by whatever they want; it's really none of my business. I'm offended by people who I think are too easily offended, but it turns out nobody gives a damn, which is as it should be.

It is my BODY. If we all treated each other with basic human respect it would be impossible to be offended by someone else's body. The very idea of being offended by someone else's body is ludicrous to me. Regardless, it is not my job to protect people's delicate sensibilities. Hey look, over there! It's a bunch of other stuff you could look at!

4. Because hypocrisy is an ugly thing. It always seems like the same group of people who are telling me I should exercise to lose weight are offended by my body in a swimsuit. While I would prefer they just shut up, I insist they choose: You can't complain about my weight and then complain about what I do to stay fit.

5. Because it is maddening to me that the diet industry makes 60 BILLION dollars a year convincing women to hate themselves. They create fear and uncertainty by saying things like, "Swimsuit season is just around the corner, are you ready to wear a swimsuit?" Well, let's see here… Swimsuit? Check. Body to put it on? Check. Yup, I'm all set thanks. Plus I think I'll keep my money, you bloodsucking leeches!

6. Because people can already see me, so they know how big I am whether I'm in a swimsuit or jeans and a t-shirt. If they are shocked at my size in a swimsuit, they should have been paying better attention.

I realize my swimsuit preferences are not everyone else's, which is awesome. Not everyone is comfortable with how much skin a swimsuit shows, regardless of their size. Here are some more ideas to help you stop obsessing and start having fun in the sun (or the oh-so-flattering fluorescent glow of the overhead lights at the gym).

1. Alternative Swimsuits. These are often created for women who want to keep specific religious clothing guidelines or who just want a more modest look. A quick Google search will turn up several options.

2. Fabulous Cover ups: If there's a particular part of your body that you prefer to keep covered for whatever reason, an (aptly-named) cover-up might be just the thing.

3. Safety in numbers. Go with a group of people who make you feel good about yourself. Focus on the fun and not on whatever body insecurities you might have. Think about how fantastic your body feels when you are swimming, or going down a water slide, or splashing in the waves.

4. Reality check. One of my favorite quotes is by Mark Twain: "I've had thousands of problems in my life, most of which never actually happened." When I'm worrying about something, I try to remember I am wasting energy on something that is not actually part of reality. So instead I…

5. …Expect the best and plan for the worst. Think about what your true fears are about going out in a swimsuit. Write them down and create a plan to deal with each of them.

Afraid people will say something mean to you? Create some scripts and practice them until you feel comfortable.

Concerned about chafing? Hie thee to Google and read up on the various lotions and powders that can help, or look into swimsuits that can help.

Worried people will talk about you behind your back? Maybe get over that. I actually think that's the best possible outcome, because frankly I don't want to hear it anyway.

In the end, of course, it's your choice. For my part, I'm not willing to allow my options for fun, activity, and movement to be controlled by what other people might think or say. If my own fears or insecurities are getting in the way, I try to find a way over (modest swimsuit), under (cover up), or through (screw this, I'm wearing a bikini) the fear and insecurity, because I've found very often the pure joy lies just on the other side.

Spanx

First, I know I'm treading on dangerous ground here as I have friends who swear by their Spanx. I'm not trying to tell anyone else how to live. If you want to wear Spanx, I fully support you. Are we good? Excellent, let's continue:

Have you seen the Spanx marketing? It says, "Spanx started with $5000 and a dream – to make the world a better place…one butt at a time!"

Big fat fail over here! My world is a better place when I can freaking breathe. My world is a better place when nobody is trying to convince me that making myself into a human sausage will make the world a better place.

Then I saw the picture on the back that showed a woman cooking in Spanx and an apron, a woman crossing a finish line wearing only Spanx, and a – my personal favorite - woman carrying a man down a ladder out of a burning building, in high heels, Spanx and nothing else, walking down the ladder facing forward, like it was a staircase.

Are you kidding me with this crap? Let's examine our three examples:

Cook a meal: If you happen to be cooking me a meal in the hopes it will get you laid, congratulations, you've got an excellent strategy there. If after that meal we find ourselves naked, and your body is suddenly a different size and shape than it was a minute ago, I'm going to think that's weird and it will probably kill the mood. Just sayin'.

Win a Race: This one kills me - this woman appears to be running in high heels without a bra, beating people who have absolutely the worst running form I've ever seen, and has been awarded her medal WHILE breaking the tape at the finish line.

Put Out a Fire: First of all, I hate to nitpick (ok, no I don't) but the girl in the high heels and compression undergarments is not putting out a fire – she is defying gravity and any modicum of ladder safety in her snazzy underpants, leaving the fire raging behind her. Second, I have to wonder how female firefighters feel about this portrayal. Third, I think I might rather fend for myself than deal with a rescue attempt by someone whose attention is on whether or not she has a muffin top.

If you want to wear Spanx, then awesome – rock those bitches. But don't try to make it an issue of my self-esteem by attempting to convince me that I will somehow be better or, even more ludicrously, make the WORLD a better place if I use super-tight underwear to temporarily change the shape of my body. You can sell a false sense of self-esteem somewhere else; I'm all stocked up with the real stuff here.

Worse than Spanx

I received the following e-mail:

Subject: A Shapewear Challenge

Body:

Hi Ragen,

I hope this finds you well. My name is Nina Lxxx and currently I am interning with Sassybax for the summer. I came across your blog post about your displeasure with Spanx, and couldn't help but notice all of the reader comments that went along with it. We would love to challenge you to try our shapewear products, and let us know what you think! … Here at Sassybax, we are committed to solving real women's problems such as muffin top or bra bulge. We would love to send you some samples to try out and see what your reaction to our product is.

All the best,

Nina

"We are committed to solving real women's problems such as muffin top or bra bulge" You. Cannot. Be. Serious.

If they are trying to convince me that calling these things problems when we live in a world with issues like hunger, poverty, racism, homophobia, and spousal abuse, they are barking up the wrong fat girl. I think marketing like this is the real problem and muffin top and bra bulge are pretend problems created by the shapewear industry in an attempt to steal our self esteem, cheapen it, and then sell it back to us at a profit.

And really, challenge? I am a three time National Dance Champion. That is a challenge. Wearing underwear? Not so much.

I would never challenge Nina to stop wearing shapewear because I absolutely respect everyone's right to choose what they want to wear. The issue is that she targeted me because I said publicly that I was happy with my body without Spanx. Her goal was to change that, make me scared of "muffin top" and "bra bulge." Had she succeeded, she wouldn't have just sold me some underwear; she would have chipped away at my hard-won self-esteem.

And it seems the intern doesn't fall far from the tree. I went to the Sassybax website and found this gem from the "about us" section.

"Fear is a great motivator," said Amanda [creator of Sassybax]. "A few years ago, when fashions got slimmer but I hadn't, I suddenly became afraid for the first time of looking my age."

So rather than work on her body image issues, Amanda chose to sell them to all of us!

Then I read her biography and was stunned, saddened, and sickened:

"Shortly after my 31st birthday, I re-entered college and finished my degree with a BA in Psychology. I earned my Master's Degree in Clinical Psychology and became a therapist. My main objective was to help women with an issue I had now come to know intimately, self esteem.

I have created Sassybax as a way of helping women look and feel more confident and comfortable in the fashions they love.

Sassybax gives women the freedom of a more natural non-restrictive kind of support. The stretchy smooth microfiber moves and breathes with your body, allowing you the freedom of being more of who you are. Now isn't that where self esteem comes from?"

I don't think I've ever read anything that made my skin crawl this much. It's so slick that it would be easy to miss the manipulation: "I'm a therapist and an expert on self -esteem. I think that to feel better about yourself you shouldn't work on your self-esteem, you should buy my underwear." Allison, if that were true, it would be called underwear-esteem.

What I'm saying here is that if someone or something is making you feel bad about your body, ask yourself if they are trying to sell you something.

Dressing for Your Body Type

"Part of the /point/ of clothing, when thoughtfully chosen, is to enhance/disguise/manipulate the appearance of our body shape."

I saw this quote in a comment on something I had written and it irked me, including and especially the emphasis on the word "point" as if I were an idiot for missing it, and the inclusion of the word "thoughtfully" to indicate that those of us who would dress for any other reason are thoughtless.

I beg to differ. So might monks, triathlon participants, and Weinerschnitzel employees. Of course, considering the roughly elebenty gabillion articles that exist at any one time in the magazines about dressing for your body type/to hide your flaws/to look 10 pounds lighter, you'd think nuns wear black because it's slimming. Sadly, this is one of these situations where someone has confused their own experience with everyone else's.

The point of clothes is whatever the wearer chooses. Clothing may be chosen:

- to enhance/disguise/manipulate a body
- to cover a body
- to show off a body
- because someone liked the print
- to be in fashion
- to rebel against fashion
- because it was clean
- because it smelled mostly clean
- because they liked it
- because it fits their company's dress code
- because it will protect them in a dangerous situation
- because they could afford it
- to please their mother
- to piss off their mother
- to express themselves
- to deal with temperature extremes
- and many more…

People may choose clothing from every point at this list, for different reasons at different times, and in different circumstances. There is no law that says clothing has to meet some criteria of being "flattering" (where flattering means thinner or closer to the societal stereotype of beauty.) If I like the idea of wearing a very clingy and bright horizontally striped tube dress, you can believe I'll be rocking that dress. Don't like it? Then take the advice that the band Chicago gave us in the 80's and "Look away, baby. Look away."

As always, other people are the boss of their enhancing, disguising, manipulating underpants and I am the boss of my adorable cotton pink polka-dotted ones, and that is as it should be.

Surviving the Biggest Loser Era

I think one of the most challenging things about the time we live in is that supposed health experts are comfortable prescribe to fat people what they would diagnose as an eating disorder in thin people. I should know – I behaved exactly like the people on The Biggest Loser, working out 8-10 hours a day and severely restricting my calories. But nobody put me on TV or gave me money. They put me in the hospital and gave me an Eating Disorder Diagnosis.

Is Jillian Michaels an Abusive Idiot?

Jillian Michaels got famous as "the mean trainer" on The Biggest Loser. She bills herself as "America's Toughest Trainer." I watched a video on YouTube in which she screamed the following at the people she was training:

- I'm bored with the pathetic story!
- If you quit on me again, you go home and no one is going to chase you! No one!
- You're not getting it here (pointing to her head) that's for G*#D#@* sure!
- Get on the F$#&ing treadmill!
- You're not acting strong, you're acting pathetic!
- Any time you lay down I want you to think Dead Father, that's what I think!
- Get. On. The. Treadmill. Now! (Pounding the treadmill to punctuate each word)
- Get the F*#k up!

The Domestic Abuse Project defines abuse as a systematic pattern of behaviors in a relationship that are used to gain and/or maintain control and power over another. More specifically they go on to say:

Emotional abuse includes:

- cursing, swearing and/or screaming at you
- attacks on self-esteem and/or insults to your person (name-calling, put-downs, ridicule)
- controlling and/or limiting your behavior
- using the difference in physical size to intimidate you
- criticizing your thoughts, feelings, opinions, beliefs and actions
- telling you that you are "sick" and need therapy

Huh.

Jillian justifies treating people this way because she claims she is saving their lives. It's "for their own good," as we fat people so often hear when someone treats us poorly. Even if we ignore the fact that no science supports this point of view, it seems to me it's more about her feeding her ego and feeling superior than it is about helping people.

I also find it interesting that while she preaches "natural weight loss" through "sweat and hard work," she has been the subject of at least three lawsuits against weight loss products she is paid to endorse including a diet pill whose tag line is "America's Toughest Trainer Makes Losing Weight Easy."

Abused people have to do a lot of work to regain their mental health, and some never fully regain it. Since there is no reason to abuse fat people in the first place, there is no reason for us to have to work very hard to regain our mental health, or risk never getting it back. Stop the abuse.

Ninety Pound Fatty?

I got a pop-up window for the "Jillian Michael's Weight Loss Plan." It was one of those deals where you enter your current height and weight and your goal height and weight, click continue, answer some questions, and then get sold stuff.

Of course the ad activated my eye-roll reflex but as I started to close it I suddenly wondered – what would happen if I gave answers that indicated I might be at risk for, or suffering from, an eating disorder? My general impression of Jillian Michaels is that she is an ego-maniac who will do anything for a buck (remember those endorsement lawsuits?) and doesn't particularly care about anyone's health. This seemed like an opportunity to see how responsible she is in her practice. And so I began my research.

I typed that I am 5'7, weigh 120 pounds, and my goal weight is 90 pounds. BMI is a crap measurement but just in case you're curious, that would give me a BMI of 14.1 – "very underweight." For perspective, a BMI of 17.5 is considered an "informal indicator" of anorexia nervosa. I also told it I liked every kind of exercise and had every kind of negative food issue.

The page that came back said my "reasonable weight is 121-153 lbs". Note that the current weight I gave it is LOWER than the lowest reasonable weight. But it lists my goal weight as 90 pounds, no problem, and then gives me the beginnings of my weight loss program. Later on e-Jillian makes sure to tell me that because of different body types there is a 10 pound leeway in both directions (remember my goal was still 21 pounds less than that) and that, "No, not everyone has big bones." Thanks, Jillian!

Then she goes on to tell me her triple-threat plan to getting me to my unhealthy, unrealistic goal weight.

Researcher that I am, I became curious as to how far I could take it. It turns out that 5'7 and 90 pounds is the lowest it would let me enter. At a weight under that amount I got a red message that said "enter a realistic goal weight." Further research showed 90 pounds is the bottom limit for every height I checked. Apparently, whether you're 4'10", 5'7" or somewhere in between, Jillian is okay with you weighing 90lbs.

My favorite phrase in her ad is: "I'm going to help you lose weight so you look and feel healthier!" Notice she doesn't say I will actually BE healthier, just that I'll look and feel this way. I'm guessing that's because she preaches caloric deficit dieting which we know has a scientifically abysmal success rate. However, she does take the time to give me misleading information about the correlations between upper body fat and heart attacks. Good use of time and typing there, Jillian.

Even with her cute customized graphics and *hilarious* puns (apparently I'm an apple but I can "pare down...") I find this really irresponsible. I think anyone who works for people's health should make it their priority to consider both mental and physical health and do everything that they can to assist clients in fostering a healthy relationship with food and their body. Measured by that ruler, Jillian falls far short.

Why people allow themselves to be treated so poorly by this woman I will never understand, but as always I'm happy for people to choose whatever life experience they want. I just suggest you think twice about following someone who, a preponderance of the evidence suggests, cares this little about what she is putting out into the world or what effect it might have on people.

Skinny Bitch, Meet Fat Bitch

There was a book on the New York Times Bestseller List called *Skinny Bitch.* The marketing quote for the book is: "If you can't take one more day of self-loathing, you're ready to hear the truth: You cannot keep shoveling the same crap into your mouth every day and expect to lose weight."

One of my roughly two million problems with this is that it assumes:

1. The food someone is eating is the cause of their current weight
2. Weight loss will cure self-loathing
3. The information they are giving is true and will work (Spoiler: they are pushing vegetarianism)

Based on the best science available, there is only a miniscule chance these assumptions are correct.

But that's not my biggest problem. My biggest problem occurs on the "Praise" page of the website:

"What makes this diet easy to swallow is the book's tough-love attitude — part best-friend counsel, part drill-sergeant abuse and a dash of sailor mouth, wrapped in a pretty chick-lit package." — *iVillage, Diet & Fitness*

Wait…did you just say abuse makes the diet easy? Are you freaking kidding me right now? Gosh, what other "medicine" could abuse help go down? Maybe we should start water boarding people who want to lose weight and haven't succeeded. Apparently as long as it's in a "pretty chick-lit package," we're all good.

Abuse doesn't make the diet easy, abuse makes the diet abusive. Fat people are not in need of abuse. Nobody is. Ever.

"This book is an absolutely hilarious read because the authors treat you like they know you well. They yell at you, they insult you and they call you some very nasty names. But since they are giving out their strongly-held beliefs and advice on living a healthy lifestyle — and you know in your heart they're right — it is refreshingly in-your-face funny." — Cathy Mathias, *Florida Today*

Screw that. Being yelled at, insulted, and called very nasty names isn't "hilarious" and "refreshing." It's abuse. See my previous comment.

This seems like just another situation where someone's ego and sense of superiority has run amok all over fat people "for our own good."

I state my strongly-held beliefs and advice on living a healthy lifestyle all the time, but I've never had to insult my readers or call them nasty names to get it done. That's because I think health includes not just physical health but mental health, and because I'm not an ego-maniacal idiot who gets my jollies from making people feel bad about themselves.

Steve Siebold REALLY Needs Your $16

Pro tip: If someone is trying to convince you to feel guilt, fear, or shame, you should immediately ask yourself "What are they trying to sell me?"

Meet Steve Siebold.

Fat Talk Free Week is a project started by the Tri-Delta sorority. Now on at least 35 college campuses, urging people during that week to just say no or "no comment" to any mention of weight, size, shape, or any other kind of Fat Talk. In the middle of Fat Talk Free Week, Bruce Serbin sent out a press release about Steve Siebold's personal mission AGAINST Fat Talk Free week. I am not kidding. Because "he's out to save as many people as he can from an early grave, but not talking about the problem is not the solution."

"Wait, who the hell is Steve Siebold?" you may be asking. Don't feel bad; I had to Google him too. He is a self-proclaimed "Mental Toughness Expert." His website lists him as a "CSP" but never explains what "CSP" means. (I found 55 meanings for those initials, none of which pertain to health.) Apparently, Steve lost some weight and wrote a book called "Die Fat or Get Tough." (I'm still not sure if he is saying that mental toughness will make me immortal or just that I should prefer to have a thin corpse, but the fact that Steve has apparently never heard of a false dichotomy is the least of my problems with this.).

I don't care whether or not Steve lost weight; I respect whatever anyone decides to do with their body. However, I have many problems with the campaign.

On the web page he says "If you're FAT [Steve likes to put FAT in all caps], this book is going to rattle your cage and make your blood boil. And it should. Get ready for a 2,000 volt cattle prod to your consciousness." Steve seriously thinks large people have somehow missed the demonstrably false myth that we are all unhealthy and, further, believes metaphorically electrocuting us is the answer. He apparently believes large people just need to feel horrible enough about ourselves and we'll be able to beat science – right after paying him $16 for his book.

He doesn't claim to have any health or fitness credentials and he is pushing a method that has been proven scientifically invalid in study after study, with an extra dose of abuse and shame, which has been proven psychologically detrimental. Again with people's ego over facts. "It's ok that I'm abusing you because I'm 'saving your life'. Now, please ignore the fact that I can't prove any of this and fork over your $16."

My main issue with Steve's Anti-Fat-Talk-Free-Week marketing campaign is that he's on a mission to make sure college students receive dangerous and harmful messages about body hatred, and to be certain that people of size are constantly reminded about the opinion (which has never been proven scientifically, and is beginning to be DISPROVEN scientifically) that fat causes health problems; and they are bad, lazy, and lack mental toughness.

I get about 386,170 negative messages about my body a year, but heaven forbid I get one week where I can actually appreciate my body or have a break from the incessant messages about body hate, because then I would miss 7,406 of those messages - and then I might not hate myself enough to buy Steve's book. You see, Steve has to convince me to let my "mental toughness" supersede my mental reasoning enough to not think this decision through, or he won't get my $16.

This campaign could be a huge problem for people who have or could develop eating disorders, a fact his publicist has admitted. If you scroll down through four pages of crap on his website, you'll find a "P.S." Literally. After his signature it says "P.S.: This book is NOT for people with eating disorders or any other physical or psychological disorders. If you think you may fall into this category, DO NOT buy this book. Instead, contact your physician and get help."

Of course. Because people with eating disorders are always able to discern they have a problem and are ready to jump on the phone and call for help. And people whose weight is affected by a physical or psychological problem are always treated really well by doctors. How irresponsible can Steve be? Could he at least open the website with that instead of this little gem:

"Do you think like a fat person? If so there's a good chance you'll DIE FAT."

Clearly he is aware of the issues his book might cause for people dealing with eating disorders; he just doesn't care enough to allow it to interrupt the flow of his marketing message, because Steve really needs our $16.

To prove he doesn't care, he is spreading this hateful, dangerous, scientifically erroneous message on college campuses. College campuses –you know, the places where up to 35% of female chronic dieters will progress to eating disorders or pathological dieting, including bulimia and anorexia, a disease that has a mortality rate 12 times higher than the death rate of all other causes of death from mental illness… I hope Steve is comfortable with being part of this deadly crisis when he cashes all of those $16 checks.

Let's get real. Most of Steve's work is as a marketing and sales coach. I think Steve saw that the diet industry makes $60 Billion dollars a year and wanted a piece of that action, so he wrote a book and started his sales and marketing machine. (Around my blog we call this "Pulling a Jess Weiner," after the woman who went to Glamour magazine under the guise of being a leader in the Size Acceptance movement and told people that the Size Acceptance movement advocates loving your body but not taking care of it in any way. What she didn't say was that months prior to this article she had trademarked the name of her new diet company). So it looks like Steve pulled a Jess Weiner. I don't think Steve knows what he's talking about and I think he knows that. I don't think he gives a crap about our health; I think he wants our $16 and figures we can clean up the mess later.

But let's pretend he really does sincerely believe what he preaches. Well, in that case, Steve has missed the point of Fat Talk Free Week by about 60 billion miles.

That's probably because Fat Talk Free Week is based on actual science, and Steve doesn't seem to be a big fan of that. FTFW's philosophy is based on research conducted by Eric Stice, a clinical psychologist at the Oregon Research Institute. Stice applied the principals of cognitive dissonance to young people. He hypothesized that, over time, a young woman who speaks and acts in a way that is contrary to the thin ideal of popular culture will eventually stop believing in that thin ideal–and thus will have less likelihood of developing an eating disorder. Stice reported a 60 percent reduction in eating disorders in high school and college students who were part of a program that critiqued the thin ideal and encouraged positive self-images. His study is not statistically significant, but it is interesting and provides more validation for eliminating fat talk than Steve has that shaming people will lead to long-term weight loss.

We know shaming people about their bodies and telling them to diet is not working. If it did, there wouldn't be any fat people. I don't care if it helps Steve get rich $16 at a time. It. Does. Not. Work.

Steve and I agree about one thing – personal responsibility. We are responsible for verifying what people say and making choices about our bodies and our health. I did the research and it will be a cold, cold day in hell before Steve gets my $16. I will continue to espouse the theory that healthy behaviors have a much higher likelihood of leading to a healthy body than emotional abuse, physical abuse, or some crazy diet. Health at Every Size is working for me- I'm happy and healthy. So I will exercise mental toughness in concert with **mental acuity** and tell Steve he can keep his emotional abuse and I'll keep my sixteen bucks.

Dancing and Weight Loss – Really Not the Same Thing

My friend to her friend: "This is Ragen. She's a bad-ass dancer. She's won National competitions!"

Friend's friend: "Keep at it, you'll lose the weight."

Me: "What the f%#k????" (Actually I said that in my head but it must have come across in my facial expression because she quickly developed an acute case of super fast talking …)

FF: "I mean, when those people go on Dancing with the Stars they lose weight and there's that Dance Your Ass Off Show and all of those people lost weight…"

I don't watch Dancing with the Stars, so it was a bit of a shock to me when I found out it's become a weight loss show. They should call it Women Wearing as Few Clothes As Possible to Divert from their Poor Technique or the Poor Technique of their Partner. Instead it's turning into "The Biggest Loser, Former Celebrity Edition." I really thought we had that covered with Celebrity Fit Club.

Then there was Dance Your Ass Off, a reality show wherein fat people learn to dance and are put on extreme diets and the only way to win is to both dance well and lose weight.

The creator of Dance Your Ass off is actress/comedienne Lisa Ann Walters. I was a huge fan of hers from her work on *Shall We Dance* where she played a fat eccentric who was a great dancer. So it actually broke my heart a little that she had jumped on the fat=fit train. Then one day she commented on my blog:

"This link came to my Dance Your Ass Off FB page and I, like you, am appalled – but, sadly, not surprised at the flourishing "size-ism" that is our last, completely acceptable prejudice. I am encouraged by voices like yours that fight. I created DYAO for that reason. I did, in fact, write a book about women and self-esteem to help combat negative body-image issues! It's funny and very empowering – I hope you get a chance to take a look, you are very inspiring. Best, LAW"

After much soul searching, I replied with this:

"First, I am such a fan of you and especially your performance in Shall We Dance. While I am honored that you would consider me inspiring, and the book looks fantastic, you are breaking my heart because I believe you that you think that Dance Your Ass Off helps to fight fat hatred. However I, who am a fat National Champion Dancer, am certain that your show and others like it are partially responsible for creating a culture where a stranger feels comfortable telling me they want to punch me until I die because I'm fat. You are an amazing actress and comedienne with a platform much bigger than mine and if I could truly inspire you, I would inspire you to encourage a focus on actual healthy habits rather than a focus on thinness that only adds to the stigma against fat people and doesn't actually increase anyone's health. Your show sends the loud and clear message that talent is not enough and health is not enough – you must be thin to win.

Thank you for the comment and very best of luck to you."

The whole dancing/weight loss thing creates an annoying problem for me. The conversation I opened with is not rare. Most people would be shocked at how many times someone appends a compliment of my dancing with "how much weight have you lost?" I understand some people think these go hand in hand but to me they are so different it's like someone telling an artist, "Wow, that's a beautiful painting. Had you considered a boob job?" Non sequitur and inappropriate at the same time.

Let's talk about what these people know in this situation. They have watched me dance, and they thought I was talented. They complimented me. Excellent logical thought process. And thank you for the compliment.

They watched me dance, they thought I was talented; they see I'm fat. They asked me how much weight I've lost. Pull the brakes and back up the logic train; we had a passenger fall off!

I haven't lost any weight. I am not trying to be thin. This is not the kind of thing to guess about. Now I'm irritated and the person who made the comment is embarrassed. This could all be avoided by focusing on what's in front of us. They don't know anything about my weight or my health, or my intentions for either, by watching me dance. They do know whether or not they think I'm a good dancer, so let's keep our eye on the ball here and stick with what we know.

The Real Biggest Loser

It's not just Jillian; everything about this show is a travesty:

What I can't believe more people don't realize is that they haven't proven this extreme behavior is necessary. The Biggest Loser contestants admit they haven't been practicing healthy habits. Does anybody but me wonder what would happen if they just made a few healthy changes to their lives; for instance, ate more vegetables, did some kind of enjoyable movement for about 30 minutes five or so days a week. What would their health look like at the end of 16 weeks? Until a show that does that is on the air, I fail to be impressed with a show that physically and emotionally abuses people in the name of better health.

Time and again I see people encouraged by "health professionals" to ignore their bodies' signals on the show – signals like pain, injury, exhaustion, and hunger. What if they started treating their bodies like friends instead of like limitations to be overcome? Our bodies give us feedback for a reason, and I'm guessing we'll be in much better health if we work with our bodies and listen to what they have to stay instead of treating them like a nuisance.

The contestants spend 16 weeks eating extremely restrictive diets and exercising 5 or more hours a day. Contestants have lost 100 pounds in seven weeks and 34 pounds in a single week. They have talked about being forced to ignore doctor's orders and dietician's recommendations by their "trainers." We glorify and reward behavior that can set these people up for a lifetime of disordered eating and a severely dysfunctional relationship with food and their bodies. Contestants have regained all of their weight and ended up in treatment for eating disorders.

Because it's a game and there is a ton of money on the line, people do things that are really unhealthy and are often considered signs of disordered eating to win: Becoming dehydrated in order to lose extra weight (the first season winner, who has now regained almost all of his weight, admitted to dehydrating his body until he urinated blood.) They also over-hydrate when they have "immunity" and want to save their weight loss for the next week. Binge eating donuts are part of a challenge, followed by trying to burn all the calories off with super intense exercise. There's the famous "last chance workout" where people push beyond all reasonable boundaries to lose that last bit of weight, and instances of people chewing massive amounts of gum in lieu of eating. The list goes on and on. If you don't see what's wrong with this, I think you need to step back and get some perspective.

The show perpetuates the idea that your self-esteem should come from fitting into the cultural idea of beauty. The trainers make it unacceptable for someone to like their body and be on the show solely for health reasons. I stopped watching completely when self-proclaimed "life coach" Jillian Michaels told a contestant his weight made him miserable. He disagreed, telling her he was happy, had a great wife, great kids and a great life and just wanted to be healthier. Jillian would not let that go. She started to berate him, insisting he was miserable until he finally said he was. Jillian was triumphant. Is this show about making people healthy, or is it about satisfying Jillian's ego? She had an opportunity to leverage his already high self-esteem to help him through the difficult process she created, but instead she felt the need to try to break him down so she could build him back up in her image. This behavior is utterly unacceptable for someone who claims to be a health professional and life coach.

These contestants are being set up for a self-esteem crash. They are taught by the trainers that their self-esteem is contingent upon weight loss, and is not intrinsic. They are encouraged to believe nobody will want to date them unless they are thin. They aren't even encouraged to derive self-esteem from the accomplishment of finishing the program. They are taught they should have self-esteem and be deserving of love only because they have become thin. What happens if they gain back their weight (as statistically a vast majority of them are likely to do)? Why can't we tell people the truth – that they are inherently, intrinsically worthy; that they should have high self-esteem because they are just awesome, without having to try at all.

There are so many people who lose on this show; it's hard to choose the biggest:

Is it the trainers who become ego-maniacs trying to justify their existence through their clients' suffering rather than nurture and assist them?

Is it the contestants who put themselves through a human experiment the likes of which a researcher could NEVER get approval for?

Is it the viewers who watch the show and buy into the idea that they can only have self-esteem and be worthy of love when they are thin?

Is it the people who try to mimic the show and become frustrated when they don't lose 100lbs in 7 weeks, or trigger an eating disorder trying?

There may only be one "biggest loser," but in the end everybody loses with this show. I'm always a little amused when people say I'm crazy for choosing to focus on healthy behaviors instead of weight loss. I think I'll stick with a sane plan that makes sense, thanks.

I think to survive the "Biggest Loser Generation" we have to remember that good television and good health are simply not the same thing. A few years ago I was contacted by some people who wanted to do a reality show about happy healthy fat people. They used my story to shop the show but it didn't get picked up because "Nobody cares about happy healthy people of any size living their lives." It's true, we don't want to watch reality shows about relationships that are going great, or friends who live together in a house and don't fight, or fatties who are happy and healthy. As a fat person in a thin-centric society we face a problem that many civil rights movements before us have faced – we rarely get to see ourselves represented in a positive light in the public discourse. We are on billboards advertising stomach amputation, we are on infomercials as "before" shots. We are on the Biggest Loser getting abused and partaking in the exact same behaviors that we send thin people to eating disorder treatment for. We are encouraged to blame every problem that happens to us on our fat, and so the message is that we won't have any more problems if we are thin. Ask a thin friend if that's working out for them.

We are not responsible for being good television, and so we can opt out and instead live a happy, healthy life, making choices that make sense to us instead of what generates the best Nielson Ratings.

Stand Back! I'm Going to Try Science

Research can be a tricky thing. A lot of this has to do with the fact that we've become much more slack about our use of scientific method. Rather than rigorously testing a theory on specific samples with well controlled variables to draw reliable conclusions, it's very likely the studies you see today have cut corners and done just enough to say their data "suggests" their conclusions, which are often foregone.

This is significant because, as you're about to see, in a 24-hour media cycle hungry for news, "suggests" and "likelihood" are often enough for the media to go to print with headlines that say "proves" and "shows," As a result, the information we get is often either misconstrued, misapplied, or just plain wrong.

The *Nutrition Journal* published a review of studies used to prove that dieting works by Lucy Aphramor called "Validity of claims made in weight management research: a narrative review of dietetic articles," Here are some of the findings:

[studies included] claims of non-specific 'health benefits' which are not substantiated.

It appears that beliefs about weight and health acquire a truth status so that they circulate as intuitively appealing 'facts', immune from scrutiny and become used, and accepted by editors, without supporting references.

Dietetic literature on weight management fails to meet the standards of evidence based medicine.

Research in the field is characterized by speculative claims that fail to accurately represent the available data.

Dr Linda Bacon and Lucy Aphramor, R.D., published a review called "Weight Science – Evaluating the Evidence for a Paradigm Shift." They found that "While it is well established that obesity is *associated* with increased risk for many diseases, causation is less well-established. Epidemiological studies rarely acknowledge factors like fitness, activity, nutrient intake, weight cycling or socioeconomic status when considering connections between weight and disease. Yet all play a role in determining health risk. When studies *do* control for these factors, increased risk of disease disappears or is significantly reduced."

There are many things to look at in a study including sample size and extrapolatability, method, drop-out rate, control of variables, and source of funding, just to name a few.

Let's take a diet study for example:

"Behavioral correlates of successful weight reduction over 3y," from *The International Journal of Obesity* (2004, volume 28, pages 334-335)

This study was referenced by a commenter on my blog as proof weight loss works. I researched it, and it turns out it gets cited a lot as proof of the efficacy of weight loss.

There are many interesting things about this study:

- "Success" is defined as "weight loss of 5% or more from baseline" over three years. So if a 5'4" person who was 350 lbs. loses 17.5 pounds and now weighs 332.5 lbs, this study calls them a success, despite the fact that they are still considered "morbidly obese" on the BMI scale.

- Other studies have shown that 95% of people gain their weight back within 5 years, so this study gave itself a two year efficacy cushion.

- The study had a 77% dropout rate. And they didn't found out why people dropped out. One reason could certainly be that they followed the strict guidelines, didn't lose weight and so quit the program.

- In total, only 198 out of the initial 6,857 people actually obeyed the seven required diet restrictions. Forty percent of those "elite dieters" failed to lose even 5% of their body weight. So, about 119 of 6,857 (1.7%) actually followed the diet and lost 5% of their body weight. Unless they were only slightly overweight to begin with, based on their own measure that amount of weight loss would have little to no affect on their "health". But experts regularly cite this study and imply that the other 99.983% of people clearly just lacked self-control.

Correlation vs. Causation

On my first day in my first research class our teacher made us say, "Correlation never ever never ever never ever implies causation" 10 times. After that we said it at the beginning and end of every class for the full semester. There is a reason why it's so important--it is the most basic tenet of research. The problem with correlational research is that it only proves things happen at the same time. It does nothing to prove that one thing causes the other, and if you can't prove the cause, you don't know the cure. When it comes to research around weight and health this means that, even if correlation is present, we have to leave room for possibilities other than just assuming weight causes the health problems.

- The weight issue and the health issue could both be caused by a third factor

- They could be unrelated and so losing weight would just mean they would just have the same problem in a smaller body.

- The health problem could be causing the weight and weight loss would either do nothing or could even exacerbate the problem.

- They could be caused by two different things and then neither issue is treated properly.

- They could both be side effects of a behavior, so a behavior change may help the health problem but not change the size of a person's body. Unfortunately, that person may be labeled a "failure" because, even though they reversed their health problem, they "failed' to change their weight.

These are just a few possible scenarios. I'm not saying a causal link is impossible; I'm saying it's not proven and nobody seems to be too worried about finding out because they are too busy yelling "IT'S YOUR FAULT FATTY!! EAT LESS AND EXERCISE MORE!!" I've heard far too many stories of people who received poor medical care because their doctor thought weight loss was a cure-all.

The media does an abhorrent job of researching stories about weight and health before they spread them far and wide, so a study where 3% of children lost weight finds itself on CNN with the headline "Say Goodbye to Obesity." The CDC retracted their statement that 400,000 deaths per year were caused by obesity.

The retraction admitted there were less than 30,000 deaths that could be connected with obesity and they admitted "the link was probably weak," but the media continues to report 400,000 deaths a year are caused by weight– which not only ignores the retraction, but also the fact that nobody ever claimed causality except the media.

There is a great deal of evidence that runs counter to the mainstream belief that you can't be healthy and fat. People are running around acting like they know the answers when they don't and that is putting the health obese people at risk due to improper medical care.

There are healthy obese people, and there are no fat-people diseases - thin people get all of the diseases correlated with obesity. Therefore, being thin can neither be a certain preventative nor a certain cure. I think we need to stop looking at weight and start looking at health. We have the ability to evaluate health with everything from blood pressure cuffs to blood panels to VO2 Max scores, so there's just no reason to look at someone's size and make guesses about their health. That's just cheap, lazy medicine. And when we continually repeat that weight is the "reason" for health issues, it gives thin people a dangerously incorrect message that they are healthy as long as their bodies remain within a specific height/weight ratio.

Health is multi-dimensional; it's a combination of genetics, access, environment, stress, and behaviors. Telling people to lose weight to be healthy is telling them to do something nobody can prove is possible for a reason nobody can prove is valid. I have a problem with that. I don't think health is a moral, societal, or personal obligation, but I do think if someone wants to be healthy, the best chance they have is to practice healthy habits. (Actually, statistically, the best chance is to be born to wealthy parents with good genes in a city where they have access to robust health care but I assume if you're reading this book then that opportunity has either come to fruition or passed you by.)I do not see how it makes sense to blame everything on a ratio of weight and height and recommend body size solutions for health issues. We have health interventions that do not include weight loss that we give to thin people for all the same diseases that we blame on obesity. Why can't we give fat people those same interventions?

Confusing correlation and causation is what leads healthcare professionals to tell fat people the solution to all of their health problems is to give their body less food than it needs in an effort to change their height/weight ratio. This is despite a marked lack of evidence that changing one's height/weight ratio is even possible over the long-term, or that it will solve their problem. Isn't it a better idea to tell people that if they want to be healthy they should practice healthy habits and actually evaluate their health to check their progress?

How Much Do We Cost the Workplace?

You probably saw the headline "Obesity Costs the Workplace 73 Billion Dollars a Year." I'm ginormous and as or more productive than anyone I know, so my first thought was, "How did they get that number?" I looked up a bunch of different articles online to make sure they were all reporting the same basic thing, and they were.

So I went to the Journal of Occupational and Environmental Medicine and paid $20 for the article, which was titled "The Costs of Obesity in the Workplace."

I will attempt to elucidate. It won't be easy, because this study is a hot mess.

Let's start with some basics:

The study looked at three factors: Medical Cost, Absenteeism (not showing up to work) and Presenteeism (being at work but being unproductive). According to my spell check, presenteeism isn't a word, but according to HR it is so we're going to go with it for now.

According to the articles I read online, the study was out of Duke University. That's true– the lead author is Eric Finkelstein, an associate professor at Duke-National University of Singapore.

The study used two sources:

The 2006 Medical Expenditure Panel Survey where BMI data is self-reported, and the 2008 National Health and Wellness Survey which is a series of self-administered internet-based questions fielded by 63,000 members of an internet-based consumer panel. Every piece of information is self-reported and unverified.

The $73 billion is an estimated projection based upon statistics that were created by doing computations with statistics and estimates, and statistics of other statistics. There are issues in the collection of data, the control of variables, the use of data, and the conclusions they drew. The study authors feel the words "obesity" and "health problems" are scientifically interchangeable and they feel comfortable assuming fat people's health problems are all caused by fatness. They also utilize BMI, which has any number of problems as a statistic in and of itself, such as the fact that it doesn't take anything into account besides height and weight and it was developed by a statistician to judge relative sizes of populations and is not a health measurement at all.

It is deplorable that news agencies reported this information as true without bringing up the limitations and issues. Studies indicate obese people already make less than their peers and are being turned down for jobs based on weight prejudice. Now companies may think they have scientific proof to back up their bias. How many of them are going to pay $20 to read and understand a complicated study?

To add another layer, under "acknowledgments" it says, "This study was supported by Allergan, Inc." This is listed as an acknowledgment, which is a problem for me, because it should be listed as a conflict of interest. Why?

"Supported" here has the meaning of "funded by."

Allergan is a pharmaceutical company. They produce Botox (sweet sweet paralysis-causing neurotoxin), Latisse (it will grow your eyelashes and don't worry, that eye discoloration is probably temporary) and…wait for it…the LapBand. The item used to bind stomachs as a weight loss surgery option.

Allergan is currently using this study from the good people of Duke Singapore to convince health insurance companies to encourage and pay for lap band surgery because it's "cheaper than the loss productivity," Astonishingly [sarcasm meter at a 9 out of 10] according to this study, the cost of obesity per person was more than the cost of lap band procedures. Let me muster up some shock… Sorry – I've got nothing.

As always, may I suggest you DO NOT need to believe everything you are told is science, and DO NOT need to take "studies" personally or allow them to affect how you feel about yourself, your health, or your productivity.

Here is a more detailed breakdown for those of you who, like me, trend toward the geeky and nerdy:

Medical Expenses

The calculation of this is statistically complicated because of the data. More specifically, the data sucks. Basically they used a two part estimate that created four categories of overweightness based on the self-reported weight. "Normal weight" was the omitted reference group. They controlled for race, household income, education, insurance coverage, marital status and smoking. They subtracted the average predicted medical expenditures for obese individuals in each category from the average predicted expenditures for those of normal weight. Then they multiplied that estimated number times the number of people in each category and added them up and extrapolated based on an estimate of obese Americans.

Problems:

First of all, notice the number of times the words estimate, average, and predicted appear in that explanation. If I had more free time I would be doing a word count to give you an exact percentage of the number of words used in this study that essentially mean "um, maybe, I guess…"; there are many.

They also didn't control for any genetic health issues or health issues that aren't correlated to weight. They appear to have assumed that any medical problems obese people had over and above what normal weight people had were solely due to fatness. They appear to have assumed that normal weight people's health issues weren't related to the same things that cause weight problems in overweight and obese people. That's just embarrassingly bad science.

Absenteeism and Presenteeism

This is my favorite (and by favorite I mean possibly the most egregious thing I've seen in a study.) These were measured based on a survey that asked people, "During the last seven days, how many hours did you miss from work because of your health problems?" and "During the past seven days, how much did your health problems affect your productivity while you were working?" Participants indicated their level of work impairment via a rating scale ranging from 0 to 10. Each response was assumed to represent a percentage reduction in productive work. Then they annualized and monetized the predictions using age- and gender-specific wage data from the bureau of labor and statistics.

Problems

Respondents weren't talking about how much work they missed or productivity they lost due to their weight, they were answering about their health problems. What they can reasonably conclude here is that people with health problems have more absenteeism and presenteeism than do people without health problems. The study's authors are basically substituting "obesity" for "health problems." You can do that, I guess, but you probably shouldn't do it while calling yourself a scientist.

Then they computed statistics using statistics and statistics of statistics. Dude. They used a 7- day sample to calculate a year's worth of data. Once again, they assumed any absenteeism or presenteeism over and above what normal weight people had was due to fatness. Except that overweight men reported less presenteeism than normal weight men. That was not reported in anywhere I could find EXCEPT the study itself, and they gloss over it.

If I had turned this work in for my very first intro-level freshman research methods class I would probably have failed the assignment and possibly been asked to leave the program because of specific incompetence and general stupidity. You don't have to feel bad about yourself – you are fine. Feel embarrassed for the scientists who put their name on this. I hope they are the laughing stock of Singapore.

Study – Can Fat People be Healthy?

You may have heard of the study by Kuk et. al. on the Edmonton Obesity Staging System. I'll give you the background first and then get to the interesting stuff and the swearing:

They characterized fat people's health on a 4 point scale: "stage 0, no risk factors or co-morbidities; stage 1, mild conditions; and stages 2 and 3, moderate to severe conditions."

They found:

Compared with normal-weight individuals, obese individuals in stage 2 or 3 had a greater risk of all-cause mortality and cardiovascular-related mortality. Stage 0/1 **was not associated with higher mortality risk** (emphasis mine.)

The study has limitations in terms of statistical significance (the sample was mostly middle class white people for example), much of the data was self-reported and the authors are clear that further research is necessary.

Some interesting tidbits:

Stage 0 or 1 participants were **less likely** to die from cardiovascular disease than "normal weight" individuals.

Stage 0 and 1 individuals were more likely to be physically active and eat more fruits and vegetables. Stage 0 or 1 participants were also **less likely to report engaging in weight loss practices.**

Hey isn't there a name for engaging in healthy habits and not engaging in weight loss practices? Wait a minute it will come to me…ah yes, it's a Health at Every Size perspective!!! I knew that sounded familiar!

Dr. Pieter Cohen, assistant professor of medicine at Harvard Medical School and a general internist at Cambridge Health Alliance said, "It's absolutely possible for people to be overweight or obese and healthy."

Dr. Sharma, chair for obesity research and management at the University of Alberta said "The key message is I can't tell you how healthy someone is if you tell me height or weight on a scale. I have to do additional tests for other health problems."

Then there are some things I almost can't believe about this:

The study says, "Nevertheless, these factors, together, indicate that obese patients, particularly in EOSS stages 0 and 1, may be better served if physicians promoted weight maintenance, as opposed to weight loss, as it remains to be seen whether individuals in EOSS stages 2 and 3 will benefit from weight loss."

Of course the articles that came out in news organizations said stage 2 and 3 patients would benefit from weight loss.

This is problematic because:

1. They JUST SAID weight loss attempts may well worsen health.

2. They don't know if losing weight will help these people. There is no solid proof.

3. Even if they did have proof that weight loss would help, they have no idea how to get it done. Prescribing something with an efficacy rate of 5%, especially knowing that the 95% who fail will likely end up less healthy than when they started, isn't just dumb – it's medically unethical.

4. I don't know whether to make study author Jennifer Kuk the blue ribbon loser or winner for this quote: "The ranking system helps to identify who should actually lose weight and who we are torturing for no reason"

Okay, Dr. Kuk. In addition to saying that you don't know if weight loss will help, in your study you said, "For the vast majority of obese individuals, lifestyle-based weight loss is not maintained over the long term (Wing et al. 1995). This is particularly concerning, given that weight cycling is associated with greater weight gain over time (Van Wye et al. 2007) and potentially worse health outcomes, compared with individuals who may have maintained a stable body weight (Blair et al. 1993; Wannamethee et al.2002)."

If you are fully aware that you are:

- ruining people's current quality of life by self-describedly torturing them
- under the auspices of possibly giving them better quality of life later
- all the while knowing the most likely outcome is actually worse health…

…may I gently suggest that **You're Doing it Wrong**.

Dr. Howard Eisenson (executive director of the Duke Diet & Fitness Center) totally doesn't get it, but got quoted in the CNN article on the subject anyway: "If we don't intervene now [when someone is healthy, 25 and obese], by the time the person is 35 … maybe some damage has been done and the unhealthy habits are more established."

Okay Dr. Eisenson, I need you to stay with me here. I'll type slowly: Not all obese people practice unhealthy habits; you're just making that up in your head. In fact the very study upon which you are commenting showed people who practice healthy habits and don't attempt to lose weight (thereby ignoring the advice of the Duke Diet and Fitness Center) have better health outcomes. Also, see above on your complete inability to effectively create long-term weight loss.

<u>Guessing About Health – Probably Not a Good Idea</u>

A study called "Separate and combined associations of body-mass index and abdominal adiposity with cardiovascular disease: collaborative analysis of 58 prospective studies" had the goal of seeing if BMI, waist circumference, and abdominal adiposity (how much fat you carry in your mid-section) were good predictors of cardiovascular disease.

They looked at information for people who did and did not develop cardiovascular disease to see if one or a combination of those measurements could have reliably predicted their disease outcome.

What did they find?

In their words: "BMI, waist circumference, and waist-to-hip ratio, whether assessed singly or in combination, do not importantly improve cardiovascular disease risk prediction in people in developed countries when additional information is available for systolic blood pressure, history of diabetes, and lipids."

In my words: They found that just looking at body size and shape was not worth doing if you could use actual measures of health. Which we can, and so we should.

<u>I'm Making You Fat Right Now</u>

Gotcha! You looked at the picture of me on the back cover and now you're going to eat cookies until you explode. If you are my friend in real life you should stop hanging out with me now before you weigh 2000 pounds.

I'm not making this up – it's "research" (research here having the meaning of highly questionable marketing copy).

Basically, a marketing professor and a marketing student conducted a study where they asked random people to take a survey:

Subjects were shown a picture of an "overweight" person, a "normal weight" person, or a lamp, and then asked to complete a survey. After completing the survey, the researchers asked respondents to help themselves from a bowl of candy as a thank you. "People who completed the survey that included a picture of someone who was overweight took more candies on average than people who saw either of the other two pictures."

"Seeing someone overweight leads to a temporary decrease in a person's own felt commitment to his or her health goal," the authors explain.

Explain? I do not think this word means what you think it means. That's not an explanation – that's a theory their research can't back up. It also reads as patently offensive to me because their false dichotomy suggests fat people DON'T have a commitment to health. (And for that, they can bite me.)

By this logic, I should be an alcoholic. You see, I don't drink. I just never started: I don't care for the taste; it's an expensive hobby and I have enough of those; and I don't like headaches or vomiting. But I spent a year as the CEO of a company that owns a bar, a restaurant, and a performance venue where we sold an astronomical amount of liquor. I was around people drinking CONSTANTLY. Yet somehow I managed to find the resolve to make my own choices. Which is amazing since it seems that according to the researchers I'm a big fat fatty with no will power who can't stop stuffing myself while bringing everyone around me down with me.

TIME Magazine let me WAY down by running with the headline "Why Seeing Overweight People Makes Us Eat More, Not Less."

It's not "Why" TIME Magazine, it's still "Does"; nobody has proven anything. I'm normally a fan of TIME but what the hell? Is it just a mistake, is your headline writer a moron, or do you not care about journalistic integrity?

Not to mention the "not less" part implies they thought the site of fat people would, for some reason, cause people to actually lose their appetite.

One more time: Correlation means things often happen at the same time, causation means one thing can be proven to cause another thing. Say it with me regular blog readers: Correlation never ever, never ever, never ever implies causation. The headlines are saying that a majority of people who looked at a picture of a fat person ate more candy, therefore seeing a fat person makes you eat more. You just can't do that. For example: in 2003 the month of August had the most ice cream eaten, and the most murders committed in the United States. So TIME should have run a headline saying "Why Eating Ice Cream Makes You Murder People."

WAIT...

If having fat friends makes you more likely to eat sweets, and ice cream is a sweet, and ice cream makes you murder people, then I'm not just making you fatter – I'm also making you a murderer. GET OUT WHILE THERE'S STILL TIME!!

As long as you're still here, let's talk about the study.

Who chose the pictures? Who judged what was considered "overweight"? Actual scientific studies have shown that different people have different interpretations of overweight, meaning some participants might have thought the "overweight" picture was normal weight and some might have thought the "normal weight" picture was underweight or overweight. Did they ask the participants? If not, does that bring their conclusions into question?

Were the researchers handing out surveys and candy all the same size?

Was there some other connection between the participants who saw the fat picture?

Did it matter that the pictures were all female?

The respondents were asked to "rank" the pictures (ostensibly a sham task). Rank them how? Did that affect results?

Did it matter if the researcher was male or female? (Participants may have been more likely to eat more candy from a male researcher, for example.)

- Could the researcher's (possibly subconscious) fat bias have lead them to offer the candy in a different way to those who saw the fat people?
- Did anybody see if the study was different if they just left the participants alone in the room with the candy?
- Was a control group offered celery?
- How many participants are we talking about here? Was the sample size statistically significant?

I'm also wondering how the lamp fared. Was it a skinny lamp or a fat one? Would that make a difference? Maybe everyone should get rid of any big furniture before they inexplicably polish off a gallon of ice cream. Or, if the people who saw the lamp ate the least candy, maybe those seeking to change their eating habits should carry around a picture of a lamp. Why didn't the study's authors draw conclusions about the lamp?

I don't know why people took more candy, and neither do these "researchers" (and I use the term loosely). It could have been complete coincidence; it could be because fat people have such a stigma attached to them that people see fat people, think about how their body will never match up to the ideal, and then eat candy as an emotional crutch, or as an act of rebellion. Nobody knows.

And really, what's the point of this research? With all the actual problems in the world, who in their right mind spends money to research whether looking at a picture of a fat person makes you likely to eat more candy? What are you supposed to do with this information?

Margaret C. Campbell, one of the authors of this study, is an Associate Professor of Marketing at the University of Colorado at Boulder. Her thesis was called "Perceived Manipulative Intent: A Potential Risk to Advertising" Some of her published papers include:

When Attention-Getting Tactics Elicit Consumer Inferences of Manipulative Intent: The Importance of Balancing Benefits and Investments

What Makes Things Cool? How Autonomy Influences Perceptions of Coolness

Implicit Theories about Influence Agents: Factors that Affect the Activation and Correction of Persuasion Stereotypes

Persuasion Sentry and Goal Seeker: How Consumer Targets Respond to Interpersonal Marketing Persuasion

Gina S. Mohr, the other author, is a Ph.D student in Marketing. I couldn't find out much about her. She has four connections on LinkedIn; I don't know if they have fat profile pictures – if so she'd better not keep candy around. Based on the exact same research techniques that she used in this study, I could publish an article that says "Why Getting a Ph.D. in Marketing Means You'll Only Have Four Friends,"

You know I'm all about healthy eating and movement for those seeking health. Maybe the first thing we should do on our path to health is exercise some common sense. Then again, I'm hungry – any thin people want to make an ice cream run with me? Come on, you know you wanna…

Math is Hard – Let's Blame Fat People?

The title of the report on CNN was "Say Goodbye to Obesity" It was late and I was tired, so like an idiot I clicked on it.

The gist of the report was that an experiment was published in the New England Journal of Medicine. Called "The Healthy Study," its goal was to increase health in children. It was a three-year, nationwide health program of school-based interventions. In this study, half of 42 schools adopted healthy food offerings and more PE time. The report tells us that students at the intervention schools kept their "weight down, sugar levels lowered and lowered their body fat". The program was deemed successful.

Question of the day: What percentage of difference between the two groups would you consider to be successful?

I won't keep you in suspense. The difference between the intervention schools and the non-intervention schools was 3%. Three. 3.

Let's see…get out my calculator… carry the four…. Yup, I'm right – the intervention failed 97% of the time. It's been a while since I was in school but I think you had to do a little better than 3% to get a passing grade back then. Shouldn't the video have been titled "Study a Big Giant Failure"? Or at least tempered "Say goodbye to obesity at least for the short term you lucky 3%"?

So I went to the source material and read the actual study – ready to yell at the people who created it. But they knew what was up. In the conclusion section they said "Our comprehensive school-based program did not result in greater decreases in the combined prevalence of overweight and obesity than those that occurred in control schools. However, the intervention did result in significantly greater reductions in various indexes of adiposity. These changes may reduce the risk of childhood-onset type 2 diabetes." If you read further you find that what they were able to do was decrease BMI and insulin levels. I have explained before why BMI is a fairly crap measurement (and if it affect BMI and not obesity then it couldn't have affected BMI that much) and I won't go into it again here, but the insulin level is significant because that is an actually measure of how they have affected the children's health.

However, they were very clear the study did NOT affect obesity. Which begs the question...why would CNN call this video "Say Goodbye to Obesity?" That's a question I will probably never be able to answer. Here are some more questions I have:

First, before someone accuses me of being against healthy food and P.E., let me say I'm all for healthy food options and more P.E. time in schools. I AM FOR CHILDHOOD HEALTH. I am glad that 3% of children were helped by this.

My concern is this: If the schools and CNN are calling this a "success," what does it say to the 97% of children who did not "succeed" by the study's own criteria? What do the P.E. teachers and health teachers say to those 97%? If they are calling the study a success, aren't they calling the 97% who didn't have experience the study's desired outcomes failures?

And what's the point of focusing on weight? We can obviously measure metabolic health in kids so what not focus on that?

So What's a Fatty To Do?

When it comes to evidence-based information about our health and lives, it's always fatty beware. The media is the absolute worst. Do not look to the media for true, clear information about health, and remember your doctor may not have the best information either. Do your own reading and ask questions. Be the boss of your health underpants.

The Self in Self-Esteem

How I got my Self-Esteem Groove Back

I wasn't always the sassy fat chick with high self-esteem who is writing this. Between high school and college I developed an issue with exercising compulsively and restricting food. I saw my body as flawed, viewing signals of fatigue, hunger and pain as limitations to be overcome through mental toughness, and I was very mentally tough. I would work out 8-10 hours a day and eat 1100 calories. In the most dramatic way possible, I collapsed on a treadmill and was given an opportunity to rethink my eating and exercise plan.

My recovery from an eating disorder took a couple days of retrospection. I looked back and my life and said, "Yeah, that was not okay; I won't be doing that again." I was EXTREMELY lucky in this, it is not a typical recovery and many people struggle with eating disorders for a large part of their lives, especially if they can't afford treatment.

At that time I had very low body fat, had stopped menstruating, and weighed 135 pounds. My doctor had told me that an appropriate weight for me was 120. So there I was, in the hospital nursing multiple stress fractures and starving TO DEATH, and 15 pounds "overweight". That was my first inkling it was the charts were wrong, not me. But then things got worse. My metabolism tanked and I gained weight extremely rapidly – almost 100 pounds over about 5 months. I was being treated for an eating disorder and simultaneously being told by doctors that I needed to lose weight.

I realized my previous behaviors weren't okay, and I wasn't going back. But I was being told by my doctors that being overweight meant a host of health problems, and I was determined to be at a healthy weight.

The one thing I felt "sure" of at the time was that I could not be trusted to make choices about my food and exercise. I thought having an eating disorder and then getting fat was proof that I should outsource my food decisions. So I let Weight Watchers, Jenny Craig, NutriSystem, Slimfast, Dexatrim, Medifast, Quick Weight Loss Center, and a host of other programs tell me what to eat.

Doctors told me that these programs would work if I just tried hard enough, and I believed them. Even though I wasn't able to maintain the weight loss over time, I just kept trying harder and harder. Then came the end of the line: I had been on one of these programs for six weeks – eating less than I had with an eating disorder, not exercising per their instructions, and gaining about one pound a week. I went in to tell them I was going to quit, and they made me go into a little office with a big poster about not quitting (you know the one – with a kitten on a rope…).

The woman started flipping through a binder with pictures of fat women. She said, "You may not know it – but this is what you look like. These women are going to die alone eating bonbons in front of the TV for the rest of their lives. Is that what you want? Aren't you tired of hating your body?"

A couple of things happened. First, I thought "*That*'s what I look like?" I was shocked because in my own mind I looked way worse than those women. I found the women in the pictures attractive. I didn't assume they were single. And the diet lady was right, I was really tired of hating my body. It was exhausting and it never made me any healthier or thinner. I started to wonder: If I felt that way about their bodies, why couldn't I think those same things about myself?

So I created a two part plan. Part 1 – I would learn to love myself and my body just as we were. Part 2: I would do the research and learn the best way to lose the weight so I could be healthy.

I wanted to actually love my body. To develop a relationship with my body where I treated it like a dear friend instead of a limitation.

I'll skip to the end. I achieved part 1 – found I loved myself and my body - discovered my self-esteem. I was happy, healthy, and could do all of the things I wanted (I'll tell you how I did it in a minute.)

Then I started exhaustive research about intentional weight loss to find the best way to get to a "healthy weight." That's when I learned no weight loss method ever tested had shown success for more than about 5% of people. I was shocked because I had assumed, based on how aggressively weight loss is sold, it must have a ton of research backing it up. But the - almost impossible for me to believe - truth was, and is, there just isn't any. Based on the evidence I decided on a Health at Every Size approach that focused on healthy habits rather than body weight.

So here I am, and I'm going to tell you how I did it. But understand, this isn't just a fat girl story. Statistically 8 of 10 women are dissatisfied with their bodies. And it's not just us – it's our daughters. Men and boys are starting to show higher levels of body dissatisfaction. About 95% of children live in a home where at least one parent is dieting 100% of the time. In a study, third and fourth grade girls stated they would rather lose a parent or get cancer than get fat. Studies consistently show 95%

of attempts at intentional weight loss fail. So we are prescribing something to 67% of the population that only works 5% of the time – and we're blaming the people who fail. Forgive me if this is too bold, but may I suggest that we're doing it wrong? So…what's the alternative?

I started by deciding I was going to fix my relationship with my body. I realized I had never appreciated a single thing my body did for me because I was so busy hating the way it looked. I had starved my body, pounded it into the ground physically and still it continued to try to support me. So I can up with these three simple steps:

1. Make a list of things you appreciate about your body (your awesome hair, your beautiful eyes, the curve of your whatever, breathing, blinking, reaching, smiling, hugging etc.) This should be a pretty long list. Mine was 64 pages.

2. Start to notice the thoughts you have about your body.

Really pay attention to when you think about your body and what you think about it. When do you blame it? When do you give it credit? When do you thank it for what it does? When do you accuse it of not doing enough? When do you think it's beautiful? When do you think it's flawed. Don't judge your thoughts, just notice them.

3. Start interrupting negative thoughts and replacing them with positive ones from the list you created in step 1.

This will take some work in the beginning. You'll have to pay attention to your thoughts and make a concerted effort to replace negative thoughts with positive ones. It's okay if you replace negative thoughts about one part of your body with positive thoughts about another. What is important is any time you think something negative about your body, you interrupt that thought and replace it with gratitude. While you're at it, start looking for opportunities to proactively appreciate your body. Soon, it will become a habit.

Bonus steps:

4. Notice the things you typically don't like about your body.

5. Think of something (anything!) to like about those things.

For example, you might hate the shape of your ass – but you would have some problems if you didn't have one at all. So hey, thanks, body for having an ass where an ass is supposed to be.

You might hate your feet, but if you can walk I'll bet you enjoy that, and I'm given to understand from conversations with friends who are amputees that walking without feet is pretty difficult. So hey, thanks feet for walking; I really appreciate it.

6. Replace negative thoughts about parts of your body with positive thoughts about the same parts of your body.

Lather, rinse, repeat and start having a little gratitude for your amazing body and everything it does for you. This exercise created the biggest shift I had in the way that I related to my body and I continue to think of reasons to thank my body every day.

Once I had a positive relationship with my body it was time to work on my overall sense of self-esteem.

Typically when I hear people talk about self-esteem they are talking about how they don't have as much as they'd like. How it holds them back. Usually they talk about low self-esteem coming from childhood, or a series of life failures. They blame it on someone or something that is "else." That's how I felt.

Here's what I realized: It's called "Self-Esteem." It's not "My-Mother-Esteem" or "My-Boss-Esteem" or "Things-Always-Go-My-Way-Esteem" or "I-Don't-Have-Any-Issues-Esteem." It's Self-Esteem.

You are the only person who can affect your self-esteem. Let me define self-esteem as I see it so as not to cause confusion. To me, self-esteem is your certainty- that you know like you know like you know - that you are intrinsically amazing.

It's not the same as how you feel about yourself because you are good at your job, or because you get the approval of others, or because of your talents, abilities and successes in life. Self-Esteem is how you would feel about yourself if you were alone on a desert island with absolutely nothing to be good at.

"Self" is the operative word in self-esteem. In my experience, self-esteem isn't developed – it's discovered. It's not a process of accumulating praise or success. It's a process of letting go of criticism and failure, letting go of praise and success. Letting go of everything and ending up with just yourself. Realizing you are incredible because you **just are** – whether or not you ever accomplish anything. If today you were a crappy, wife, mother, sister and friend, then you are an awesome person having a bad day. If you are not happy with your life, then you are an awesome person who made some bad choices or had bad things happen to you. But you are still awesome.

If you don't get that, then no achievements, promotions, praise, approval, love, or success will ever be able to give it to you. And if they are able to give you a false sense of self-esteem, you are always just one failure away from not having any.

You have to get that you are amazing and worthy – at this moment, at every moment – and you don't have to do anything to have that, be that, or deserve that. It just is. Nobody can give it to you; you have to discover it, claim it, and own it for yourself, then nobody can take it away.

Then you scrape together everything you found about your inherent, intrinsic amazing-ness and you say "This is my Self-Esteem. It's mine. It's precious. You can't touch it. You can't even get near it. You can have my self-esteem when you pry it from my COLD. DEAD. HANDS." Then you move forward with the work of being the person you want to be. You love yourself first, and then you make choices and deal with life as it comes at you. It's not a magic bullet and it takes work but I have found that life is easier when I'm standing on a platform of high self-esteem.

Eat a Sandwich

The blog I wrote that first got a lot of attention was about a quick experiment I did to see how many negative messages I got about my body on a daily basis. (It added up to 386,170 negative messages a year.) While I was researching it, some of the messages I heard were:

"Fat isn't sexy, it's a fact."

"Men just don't want obese women"

"Everybody knows you can't be healthy and obese"

I don't know about you, but I don't enjoy getting those messages from society; it's frustrating and it hurts my feelings.

While perusing some "size positive" blogs, I found the following comments:

"Stick women just aren't sexy, it's just gross."

"What man would want a twig anyway?"

"It's just impossible to be healthy when you are that thin; you have to be anorexic or a drug addict to look like that."

"Real women are curvy and LOOK like women."

I absolutely understand why people in the size positive community say things like this. It's rare to see people on television and in commercials who look like us, and that can be frustrating. We're getting hundreds of thousands of negative messages about our bodies every year and we are tired, angry, and hurt. People with no health credentials feel completely justified in making assumptions about our health. Doctors make the same mistaken assumptions. It's easy to transfer our frustration onto the people who represent "the other side." Sometimes you've just taken all you can stand and you feel like you have to lash out. I get it – I really do. I've been there. That being said:

Knock it off.

Seriously.

If we want people to treat us with respect when it comes to our bodies, we should take a pass on bashing other people's bodies and it doesn't matter if they have "thin privilege" or not.

If we want people to take a good, hard look at their size prejudices, we should take a good, hard look at our own.

Health at Every Size means health at EVERY size. Size Acceptance means ALL sizes. If we insist some people are naturally larger, then it follows some people are naturally smaller. It astounds me that someone who screams "IT'S NOT FAIR!" when they are judged unhealthy because of their size would turn around and do the same thing to someone else.

I want a world of body positivity; a world where everyone is treated with respect and dignity, where everyone knows they are beautiful and receives acknowledgment of that from society. Nobody should be treated the way fat people are currently treated in our culture. Nobody. So I want change, but not if it means treating thin people like fat people are treated now. That's too high a price to pay.

I believe if you say you want a size positive world, you have to mean size positive for everyone. That means not making judgments about others based on their size, sticking up for the model being called anorexic with the same fervor you would use to defend a fat women being called lazy, and respecting other people's decisions when it comes to their bodies – even when you don't agree with them.

That's what it means to be the change you want to see in the world.

There is no excuse for these behaviors, but I've heard plenty of people try to excuse them. Typically the excuse is something like, "They have so much privilege as a thin person that it doesn't matter."

Look. The fact that people have "thin privilege" (which they typically never asked for) does not mean you can just bash them all you want. Besides, this isn't just about them. The fat community is extremely disenfranchised. Many of the people of size I talk to have internalized the oppressive messages they get from society (we're lazy, unhealthy, a drain on society, unattractive, etc.) to the point that it has become an identity for them. That's not a foundation upon which you can build a civil rights movement. It's hard to demand respect when there's a chorus of your community members still convinced they don't deserve to be treated well.

So how about we start with our own actions? This isn't the Oppression Olympics; there's no medal for being the group who has it worst. I think the most important thing we can do when we are looking for respect and equality is be examples of what that means in our day to day life.

Even if thin women's privilege protected them from the pain of comments like "eat a sandwich", "you're anorexic," "real women have curves" and other such B.S. (and I don't think it does protect them) it is still an astoundingly bad idea to verbally bash them.

Because even it doesn't hurt them, it hurts us. When we do to others what we don't want done to us, justifying it because it doesn't happen to them very often, we become a bunch of things that aren't good:

- hypocrites
- lacking in integrity
- part of a system we claim we want to end
- just as bad as everyone who has ever said anything to us about our size

This is not about **someone else's** privilege.

This is about **our** integrity.

Are you or are you not someone who believes everyone, and their body, deserves to be treated with respect? Are your actions consistent with who you say you are?

I know that fat people are hurting in our culture, and we absolutely deserve to be treated better. But I'm here to tell you that the only way out is up – you can't get out of a hole by digging, and you'll never get respect for your body and choices by disparaging someone else's.

I hope we can all get on the same page in believing that being the change you want to see definitely does not include doing to others the **exact thing** we are asking people to stop doing to us.

Trying to hurt someone else in the same way you've been hurt never works. You can't improve your self-esteem by diminishing someone else's. In the end you won't feel better and there will be two people in pain.

If you want to lash out, do something really radical, something that really takes courage: respect and find beauty in every body including your own.

Flying Fat People

Airlines' poor treatment of fat people is receiving more and more press. Famous movie producer Kevin Smith started a storm of press when he used Twitter to chronicle his experience of getting kicked off a Southwest Airlines flight for being too fat, despite meeting their policy requirements for fitting in the seat.

When it comes to charging large people more, airlines' policies go something like this: The airline is selling space. The amount of space is one seat. Space is at a premium on an aircraft and the carriers have created a price for that amount of space.

There are plenty of arguments made for changing this policy, and I'll make those in a few pages. However, since this is the policy right now and assuming that we would like to fly now, I propose the following argument that I believe will help them see the beauty in accommodating passengers of all sizes: If that is their policy then it must be applied across the board. Right now, it's ok if your legs are too long and you have to encroach on someone else's space, or if your shoulders are too wide and they overlap into the next seat. The only people who are being kicked off planes are people whose butt or torso is in someone else's space.

That's not about everyone getting their fair share; it's just about punishing fat people. Anyone who takes up more than one seat needs to pay more or it's clear discrimination. I happen to fit easily in one airline seat (sheer luck; my fat goes out in front of me and not out to the sides). The last flight I was on I fit into the seat just fine, but the tall, thin gentleman beside me had very broad shoulders and he encroached upon my space. If the airline is charging people who take up more than their fair share, this man needs to pay up as well. I am a kind, empathetic flyer and didn't complain about the encroachment – people come in different sizes included broad shouldered. However, if I had been hassled or asked to pay more, you can bet I would have been pointing this out.

Dealing with Airline Policies and Procedures

It's not you, it's them

The airlines have policies and procedures and that's fine, but you have every right to expect that they will treat you with good customer service, and that they will explain their policies clearly and apply them consistently. If they view you as an inconvenience, that's their issue, not yours. Also be aware the perpetrator of this behavior may be a jaded employee who views everyone who is not young, quiet, thin, and flying without kids as an inconvenience. That is not your fault but it can become your problem. You deserve a great experience. You and your body deserve to be treated with respect, especially when you are paying the airline for a service. There is no need to feel embarrassed about asking questions. For me, the goal of flying is to get where I'm going with my dignity, sanity, and sense of humor intact. This is how I do it:

The truth about airplane seats

The average coach airplane seat measures between 17.2 and 18 inches across, so you'll probably feel squeezed if your hip measurement is more than 36 inches. (I've read the average American woman's hips are between 44 and 46 inches and the average American men's are 38 inches, so it seems most people are pretty uncomfortable in an airplane seat.)

One thing that is less talked about but may be more crucial is "pitch" - the measurements between seats aligned vertically.

This measurement has changed quite a bit as airlines have added additional rows. Small pitches mean people aren't able to move their legs as much.

In first class, the typical pitch is about 80 inches. In coach it's usually about 31 inches. Some airlines do offer seats (typically at an upgrade price) that offer more legroom. If a person is over six feet with hips wider than three feet, they are probably going to feel very squished (that's a technical term) both vertically and horizontally.

Know your airlines

Information is power; have as much of it as you can. Create a folder or binder you take with you to the airport. Make it look professional. Keep it organized and impressive. Make sure it is easily accessible from your carry on. This will be important later.

Google

Use search terms like "Fat friendly airlines," "[airline name] oversize passengers," "[airline name] fat passenger." Print out any pertinent details and put it in your folder.

Research the airlines website

Use the search function to find information about the policy. Read the policy thoroughly and make note of any questions that you have. Print out a copy of the policy and highlight the pertinent details. Place this in your folder.

Call the Airline

This one isn't for everyone, but if you're into documentation then it's absolutely an option. When you make the call, remember your body is nothing to be embarrassed about. The people who you talk to may be embarrassed about it, and that's to your advantage. Keep the power here by remembering you are a customer asking for a clarification of a policy that may or may not exist and may or may not apply to you. The airlines have screwed this up, not us. So we should feel embarrassed for them, not embarrassed by them.

When you talk to an employee, write down the date, time, their name and title, and the details of the conversation. Ask them for general information and any questions you have about the online policy.

If they tell you it's up to the ground crew or the flight crew (and this is pretty likely), ask for a manager. Explain you are about to pay a lot of money for a ticket and that it is unacceptable to you that they can't tell you how much it is going to cost for you to fly with them.

It is very possible that you will be told to buy two tickets just in case, and then promised a refund when you get there if you don't need it or if there is an extra seat available. If you can afford it and are willing, this might be a good "better safe than hassled" option. If you can't afford it or don't want to do it, I would suggest telling the manager it's unacceptable that you should have to spend extra money because they aren't able to clarify their policy. Get the manager's name and title. Escalate the call and have this conversation again. It's possible you still won't get a satisfactory answer, but at least you'll have documentation in case you need it.

Put the details of these calls into your folder.

The goal here is to document everything you've done to make this process go smoothly in the event that you have trouble at the gate.

At the Gate

It's not fair that we fat people have to do this. But this isn't a chapter on fairness or on lobbying the airlines for better treatment (both of which are worthy activities.) This is a chapter about how to best deal with things as they are right now.

Choose: Proactive or Wait-and-See

Once you get to the gate, you have two options. You can be proactive and ask questions, or you can wait and see if you have any issues. There are pros and cons to both.

Proactive

The upside to this is that you get it dealt with early so you don't have to sit and stress about whether or not you're going to have an issue. The down side is that if you bring it up, you may be inviting trouble. If you want to go this route, go immediately to the attendant at your gate. Say, "I'm just confirming that, based on my research and my conversation with so-and-so at your airline (show your impressively organized folder), there won't be any issue with my size."

A few things might happen here:

The gate agent might say that it's up to the flight crew. I think this is crap; the policy should be known and applied across the board, and if it's me, I'm asking for a manager to clear that up.

If you don't want to ask for a manager, ask what will happen if they determine that you'll need two seats. Make sure to write down everyone's name, title, and the details of the conversation in your folder.

They might say that you are fine; in that case grab a pen and document the time, date, their name and exactly what they said. Be polite.

They might say you need to purchase a second seat. Since you've done your research, you'll already know their policy on whether they give a discount for the second seat, (some airlines do a discount, some do half price, some insist that you pay full price, some will refund your seat if there ends up being an open seat on the plane. Since they change all the time, I'm not going to list the current policies here – sorry!) You can take this time to clarify that policy and buy a second seat. You can refuse and ask for a refund. You can ask if the policy applies to thin people whose shoulders are too broad to fit in a seat. (That should lead to an interesting conversation.) You can ask for a supervisor.

If you don't have another way to get where you want to go, this situation can feel pretty powerless. They have all the cards, since they have your money for the original ticket and the ability to stop you from boarding the plane. If possible, have another option to get where you are going. If that's not possible, you'll have to negotiate whatever you can with the manager. Stay calm. Avoid calling them names or raising your voice. Try to get the manager on your team. Make it you and the manager against a problem rather than you against the manager. Show all of the due diligence in your folder and explain how frustrated you are that after all that work you're still being hassled at the gate. Explain that while you understand that it's not the manager's fault, you are a customer who went WAY above and beyond the call of duty to avoid hassle, and here you are being hassled because the airline doesn't have a clear policy. Consider negotiating an upgrade to first class.

Wait and See

This is what I do. I think it's the ground crew's job to bring up any problems before I board the plane. I don't have to ask for a seat belt extender because I brought my own (more about that in a moment). I organize my stuff immediately so that I don't have to shift around too much after the plane takes off. (I put my book, iPod, my due diligence folder, etc. in the seat pocket in front of me.) I have never had any trouble. Typically I think the flight attendant just wants to get through the flight so if they aren't personally weight bigoted and if the person beside you doesn't make a fuss, the flight attendant won't make a fuss either. I've never had an issue.

If I did, I would first explain all my due diligence. I would grab my folder, allude to the online policy and my phone call and explain that they hadn't said anything about it at the gate. I would then ask what solutions were available – is there an empty seat that I can sit next to? How about in first class? While that is going on, I would be trying to count the number of people I could see whose shoulders were too broad or legs too long to fit in their seat. If they can't quickly and quietly find a solution for me that doesn't cost additional money, I would ask the flight attendant why the policy isn't being applied across the board to include people whose shoulders are too broad or legs are too long. I would have my pen and folder out and by recording all of this information.

Again, I would stay calm and try to make it me and the employee against a problem rather than me against the employee and see what could be negotiated.

Practice makes Proud

As always, you can always take time beforehand to go over likely scenarios and practice what you will say. You can write it out if you like or just practice in your car at home or on your way to work. Be prepared and you'll have a much better chance of ending up proud of the way you behaved and the things that you said. I've found that absent this practice, I just start screaming and getting emotional and then people view me as the screaming, emotional fat girl, and that tends to be pretty ineffective. I expect the best but prepare for the worst.

Airline Tips and Tricks

BYOB – Bring Your Own Belt

Seat belt extenders can be purchased reasonably cheaply online from places like moreofmetolove.com. There are two types, conveniently named Type A and Type B. Type A are used for most commercial airlines; Type B are used predominantly for Southwest Airlines (which I would not fly for any amount of money because of their history of poorly treating passengers of size and GLBT passengers).

The Joy of the Aisle Seat

I highly recommend an aisle seat if you can get it. Not only can you lean into the aisle, but many people don't know that the arm rest on the outside of the aisle seat raises up. There's a trick to it and it's different on different planes. Often it's a button on the underside of the arm rest. You can always ask the flight attendant. Typically you have to have it in the lowered position for take-off and landing but it can make the rest of the flight way more comfortable.

Be friendly and empathetic

You deserve to be treated with respect in every interaction, including when on a plane. Realize that while it's not your fault that the seats are small, the pitch is narrow and the airline can't accommodate you properly, it's not the fault of the person sitting beside you either. Recognize that if the person next to you fits in their seat and you do not, their view is likely to (logically) be that you are encroaching on space they paid for. Demand respect, but do be empathetic. Decide if you want this to be a moment to start a dialog or you just want to get through the flight. As always, it's your choice. I often smile and say "I'll bet we both wish that the airline did a better job of accommodating passengers of different sizes." That tends to smooth things over.

Why Shouldn't Fatties Have to Pay More

It seems like every few months the news will float some story of some person who was so enraged at having to sit next to a person of size that they made a fuss, walked off the plane or whatever.

I don't know how much of a problem this really is. It might be one of those things that is used to stigmatize fat people even though it rarely comes up in real life. (Which is not to say that it doesn't cause a ton of stress for fat people worrying about it, or fat people who just don't fly because of it – I'm just saying it may be that people rarely complain.)

The main problem is subjectivity and unpredictability. You won't know the situation until you get on the plane. You may be able to fly easily on the first leg of your trip only to be told by a flight attendant that you are too fat for the second leg. Plane seats are different sizes, seat belts are different lengths. It's difficult to decide who actually "fits in a seat." A weight limit doesn't work – I'm almost 300 pounds but my fat happens to go forward rather than sideways so I fit in a seat, there are people one hundred pounds lighter than me who don't fit in a seat because they carry their weight differently. Hip and thigh measurements don't really work, for the same reason. But if we take up more space, why shouldn't we be charged more?

Again, the general argument about this goes that the airline is selling space and therefore if you don't fit in a seat you should pay extra. I do understand this argument and why there is controversy about this. The primary reason I disagree is that the airlines are selling transportation to people, people come in different sizes and shapes, and therefore I think that the airlines are responsible for accommodating their actual passengers and not just those who are a specific size. We are all paying to get our bodies from one place to another.

I've seen flight attendants bend over backwards to accommodate a tall passenger, and if someone wants to use the "tall isn't their fault but being fat is" argument (thought I don't agree with the premise), then I've seen flight attendants bend over backwards for someone wearing a cast and using crutches and, having watched the show Jackass, I know that could very well be the result of doing something incredibly foolish. At the end of the day, it's about getting bodies from one place to another. People come in different sizes, this is the size I come in, and I need to get from here to there just like everybody else who is getting on this plane.

Also, I would suggest that this is thinly-veiled fat discrimination because nobody ever says anything about men (and sometimes women) whose shoulders don't fit within their prescribed area – next time you get on a plane look at how many people's shoulders are in someone else's seat. We're also not talking about people with body odor or people who have marinated in cheap cologne and make the flight unpleasant for a couple of rows of passengers – should they be required to purchase all the seats within smelling distance?

We keep hearing how airlines are struggling financially. You would think that if more than 60% of Americans are fat then it might make financial sense to court us for our business, not treat us like we are an unbelievable pain in the ass because we have the audacity to exist, and because their attitude of covering their eyes, plugging their ears and screaming LALALALALA instead of acknowledging that we exist and working to actually accommodate us results in us bothering some tiny percentage of the 30% of people with whom the airlines actually seem to want to do business.

This is a problem, but the solution is definitely not to set some arbitrary weight at which people should have to pay extra, or to have people entering their hip measurements along with their credit card numbers when they book.

Accommodating fat people is not rocket science. Canada has a one-passenger one-ticket rule so clearly it's not impossible.

Put us in the aisle – Again - the aisle armrest actually raises. You have to keep it down during take-off and landing, and you have to squish when the drink cart comes by, but for the vast majority of the flight you can gain a lot of space.

Standby Tolerance - Choose which standby passengers get to fly based on who is willing to sit next to a person of size.

Do Not Accommodate Weight Bigots - If the person sitting next to you has their body in your seat but isn't touching you, then you may have 99 problems but a fatty ain't one, enjoy your flight. If the person sitting next to you is touching you, then welcome to the experience of millions of people taking public transportation every day, this may not be your favorite flight ever-it happens. I've been seated next to a shrieking baby, in front of a kicking toddler, near people with some serious body odor, near other people wearing half a bottle of the world's most noxious perfume. I'm allergic to cats and I spent 4 hours sitting (and sneezing) next to a woman with a sick cat in a carrier in her lap beside me. None of these were fun flights, but in each case I can empathize. Also, get a grip - it's a few hours out of your life, you don't have to spend a month on this plane. If you don't want to deal with other people in close proximity, public transportation is not for you.

Row o' Fatties - Stick all the fatties in the same rows. We'll snuggle.

First Class Fatties - This one will be controversial, but if the airlines fail to be able to accommodate passengers of size in coach, they could offer a discount to fatties who want to fly first class.

These are just off the top of my head; I'm sure that there are other solutions. I do know that the solution is not to tell fat people that they need to change their bodies; not just because nobody can prove that it's possible for the majority of people, but also because weddings, family reunions, funerals and vacations are happening now, not 50 pounds from now.

We need to start being fatties, airline passengers, and airlines together against a problem, not airlines and airline passengers against fat people. Fat people are in fact people. We're just like you, only bigger. We deserve the same ability as everyone else to buy one ticket for our one body, get on a plane, and get safely to our destination without being the subject of bullying, harassment, or bigotry because of how we look.

Won't Somebody PLEASE Think of the Children

As body-policing and inappropriate as people can be with adults, when it comes to kids they can lose their freaking minds. Suddenly people are trying to get kids to hate themselves healthy - shaming them about their weight because they believe that the ends justify the means. Even fat people can fall into this trap; they so viscerally remember how difficult it was to be a fat kid that they don't remember that no amount of this kind of treatment made them into a thin or healthy adult.

Let's examine the war on childhood obesity and see how it's going:

Michelle Obama

Michelle Obama decided to start a "war on childhood obesity" with her "Let's Move!" campaign. She said she was going to "end childhood obesity in a generation."

As part of this, both she and the President have called their own children chubby *on national television.*

She publicly put her 8 and 11 year old daughters on diets.

Despite the fact that obesity is not a disease and intentional weight loss has only a 5% long-term success rate, Mrs. Obama felt comfortable saying "This isn't like a disease where we're still waiting for the cure to be discovered. We know the cure for this…this doesn't require new technology, or, you know, new research. We have the solution in our hand."

In saying this, she set up the 95% of kids who will statistically fail to become thin (and, based on studies will have a much higher chance of developing eating disorders and lifelong issues with food and weight) for a heaping helping of bullying for being fat – because Michelle Obama says they could have been thin if they tried hard enough.

She repeatedly refers to childhood obesity as a "problem" that needs to be "fought" and "fixed."

Let's look more deeply.

Obese kids do not separate themselves from their fat. You cannot have a war against childhood obesity without having a war against obese kids. If you say childhood obesity is a "problem" that needs to be "fought" and "fixed," then obese kids hear that THEY are a problem that needs to be "fought" and "fixed."

We need to look not just at physical health but at mental health as well. I don't think stigma and shame go hand-in-hand with either. According to the US Department of Health and Human Services, hospitalizations for kids under 12 with eating disorders are up 119% between 2000 and 2011.

A study published in the April 2006 Journal of the American Dietetic Association looked at dieting as a predictor of eating disorders. The researchers at the University of Minnesota found that dieting among adolescents can predict the development of eating disorders and obesity in later years, but did not predict "normal weight" adults.

Researchers found that students who engaged in dieting were three times more likely to be overweight five years later than adolescents who did not engage in those behaviors. They were also at significantly increased risk for binge eating with loss of control as well as extreme weight-control behaviors such as self-induced vomiting and the use of diet pills, laxatives and diuretics.

According to the researchers: "None of the behaviors being used by adolescents for weight-control purposes predicted weight loss. Of greater concern were the negative outcomes associated with dieting and the use of unhealthful weight-control behaviors, including significant weight gain."

Said more simply, The least likely outcome of dieting was weight loss. The most likely outcomes of dieting were weight gain and eating disorders. Michelle Obama had access to this information six years BEFORE she started her Let's Move! Campaign.

In a separate speech about her anti-bullying initiative, Mrs. Obama said kids should have a "chance to learn and grow without constantly being picked on, made fun of, or worse...." Somehow I think using parents, teachers, health care professionals and peers to convince kids their bodies are problems that need to be fixed does not give them access to the chance to learn and grow.

In the same speech she said kids shouldn't be made to feel "afraid for being different." But it seems like she thinks kids whose bodies don't fit into a very narrow height and weight range should definitely be made to feel afraid for being different.

And that doesn't take into account the disservice we do to thin kids who aren't practicing healthy habits. When we use body size as a health diagnosis, we make the assumption that every fat kid eats too much and doesn't exercise enough and every thin kid eats and exercises the right amount. That's simply not true. All of us went to school with a kid who was thin despite never exercising and eating nothing but junk food. Oddly, we accept that there are bodies which can stay thin despite not eating a healthy diet or exercising, yet we reject the notion that some bodies don't stay thin despite eating a healthy diet and exercising. Either way, singling out fat kids means thin kids receive the message that as long as their bodies remain thin, they are "healthy" and don't have to practice healthy habits.

Lucky for this generation of kids, being told by your doctor, teachers, parents, and the First Lady of the United States that your body is unhealthy and a problem is not just charming, it's superb for your mental health and will have absolutely no future negative ramifications. It is certainly the kind of thing that gives kids the "chance to learn and grow without constantly being picked on, made fun of, or worse…" (sarcasm meter is a 10 out of 10 on this.)

While I'm on a sarcasm roll, apparently kids shouldn't be made to feel "afraid for being different" unless the difference is their size. It's okay for everything in nature – horses, trees, rocks, feet etc. - to have a wide array of sizes. But if a human body doesn't fit into a very narrow range, it should be considered a problem that needs to be fought and fixed. And do let's point that out as often as possible. It's not about being healthier, it's about being smaller and feeling horrible about yourself until you do.

Since the First Lady says we don't need any "you know, new research," let's go with some research we already have:

According to sources cited on the non-profit National Association of Anorexia and Associated Eating Disorders website:

- 47% of girls in 5th-12th grade reported wanting to lose weight because of magazine pictures.

- 69% of girls in 5th-12th grade reported that magazine pictures influenced their idea of a perfect body shape.

- 42% of 1st-3rd grade girls want to be thinner.

- 81% of 10 year olds are afraid of being fat.

So our kids don't need the First Lady's help to be unhealthily obsessed about their weight; they've got that going for them already.

While we're at it, there are some compelling reasons not to put kids (like, say, for a random hypothetical example, 8 and 11 year old girls) on diets:

Again according to ANAD:

- 91% of women surveyed on a college campus had attempted to control their weight through dieting
- 22% dieted "often" or "always"
- 35% of "normal dieters" progress to pathological dieting. Of those, 20-25% progress to partial or full-syndrome eating disorders
- 95% of those who have eating disorders are between the ages of 12 and 25.8

So maybe we could back the hell off of fat kids and be a nation that is for healthy options for kids and their parents, of all sizes, and against telling obese kids or adults that the bodies they live in 100% of the time are a "problem" that needs to be "fought" and "fixed," and waging a war on them to prove it.

I am for giving kids healthy choices, and if Mrs. Obama's program was also for giving kids healthy choices, I would be behind it 100%. I am against conflating health and weight, and singling out fat kids when it's completely unnecessary to helping kids of all sizes be health, and does nothing more than create panic, fear, poor body image, and the perfect environment for bullying.

I am against bullying. I am very happy the Obamas started an anti-bullying campaign. However, I am also against hypocrisy and I would like them to apply their anti-bullying standards to programs like "Let's Move" so they are excruciatingly careful not to accidentally encourage bullying when they intend to encourage healthy behaviors.

Our Fat Chance for Health

"Obesity Weighs Heavy On Our Health," says the headline (which always contains some kind of weight pun – so hilarious.) You cannot live in this country and not hear the message that fat is unhealthy. The diet and beauty industries spend billions of dollars spreading that message around, getting us to spend over a hundred billion dollars on their products every year.

When I look at our culture I see very little talk about health and a whole lot of talk about body size, and I think that's really what weighs heavy on our health.

BMI

Typically when people start talking about size and health, they use the Body Mass Index (BMI) as their guide. But what is it? Belgian polymath Adolphe Quetelet devised the BMI equation in 1832 as a statistical tool. It was meant to be used to compare body sizes among large populations. It was not intended to be used to judge health at all, let alone health of individuals. The BMI is a simple ratio of weight and height. As such, it doesn't take into account muscle mass or any actual indicators of health (glucose, triglycerides, blood pressure etc.) BMI only gives you a ratio of someone's height and weight. Insurance companies started using it because it was cheaper than measuring actual markers of health, and it became popular to talk about BMI as a measure of health. Soon BMI ranges were created and categorized as underweight, normal weight, overweight, and obese, and we were off to the races. So, it's not that BMI is a poor measure of health, it's that BMI is not a measure of health at all.

25 Million Americans Become Overweight Overnight

Three members of the committee responsible for reviewing the standards for obesity including BMI as a risk measurement had direct ties to pharmaceutical companies that manufactured diet pills for profit. A fourth member was the lead scientist for the program advisory committee of Weight Watchers International. Their recommendations shaved 15-20 lbs off the definition of "normal weight," which made 25 million Americans "overweight" overnight.

The CDC accepted their recommendations and they went back to their home companies with 25 million more potential customers. Headlines ran in many major media outlets: "Million of Americans Don't Realize They Are Overweight." Those articles failed to mention that those people hadn't been overweight the previous day. People who would have been considered a "healthy weight" a day ago were now told that they had to lose weight to be healthy, and were being marketed to by the very people who had made them overweight just 24 hours before.

Something that's interesting to me is that studies are starting to show that obese people who live in cultures where they aren't stigmatized do not experience the same negative health outcomes as those in cultures where obesity is stigmatized. Peter Muennig at Columbia University found that women had more physical and mental illness if they were concerned about their weight, regardless of their weight. He also pointed out that the stress of being under constant stigma was correlated to the same diseases to which obesity is correlated. So it may not be our weight but rather the stress of living in a world where we are constantly stigmatized and told that we are sick, unhealthy, unattractive and unworthy of love, or it might be something else entirely.

What's important to remember is nobody knows, and our culture is so wrapped up in our obesity hysteria that we're not trying to find out.

Does Weight Loss Work?

On the lack of evidence for the efficacy of weight loss:

"There isn't even one peer-reviewed controlled clinical study of any intentional weight-loss diet that proves that people can be successful at long-term significant weight loss. No commercial program, clinical program, or research model has been able to demonstrate significant long-term weight loss for more than a small fraction of the participants. **Given the potential dangers of weight cycling and repeated failure, it is unscientific and unethical to support the continued use of dieting as an intervention for obesity**." — Wayne Miller, exercise specialist at George Washington University (emphasis added)

On the myth that people who have lost weight eat like "normal weight" individuals:

"Geissler et al. found that previously obese women who had maintained their target weights for an average of 2.5 years had a metabolic rate about 15% less and ate significantly less (1298 vs. 1945 calories) than lean controls. Liebel and Hirsch have reported that the reduced metabolic requirements endure in obese patients who have maintained a reduced body weight for 4-6 years.

Thus, successful weight loss and maintenance is not accomplished by "normalizing eating patterns" as has been implied in many treatment programs but rather by sustained caloric restriction. This raises questions about the few individuals who are able to sustain their weight loss over years.

In some instances, their eating patterns are much more like those of individuals who would earn a diagnosis of anorexia nervosa than like those with truly "normal" eating patterns." Garner DM, Wooley SC Confronting *the failure of behavioral and dietary treatments of obesity. Clinical Psychology Review1991;6:58–137*

And from the *New England Journal of Medicine*:

"Many people cannot lose much weight no matter how hard they try, and promptly regain whatever they do lose…Why is it that people cannot seem to lose weight, despite the social pressures, the urging of their doctors, and the investment of staggering amounts of time, energy, and money? The old view that body weight is a function of only two variables – the intake of calories and the expenditure of energy – has given way to a much more complex formulation involving a fairly stable set point for a person's weight that is resistant over short periods to either gain or loss, but that may move with age. …Of course, the set point can be overridden and large losses can be induced by severe caloric restriction in conjunction with vigorous, sustained exercise, but when these extreme measures are discontinued, body weight generally returns to its preexisting level."

Mann T, Tomiyama AJ, Westling E, Lew AM, Samuels B, Chatman J: **Medicare's Search for Effective Obesity Treatments: Diets Are Not the Answer.**

"The authors review studies of the long-term outcomes of calorie-restricting diets to assess whether dieting is an effective treatment for obesity. These studies show that one third to two thirds of dieters regain more weight than they lost on their diets, and these studies likely underestimate the extent to which dieting is counterproductive because of several methodological problems, all of which bias the studies toward showing successful weight loss maintenance. In addition, the studies do not provide consistent evidence that dieting results in significant health improvements, regardless of weight change. In sum, there is little support for the notion that diets lead to lasting weight loss or health benefits."

Miller, WC: **How Effective are Traditional Dietary and Exercise Interventions for Weight Loss**

"Although long-term follow-up data are meager, the data that do exist suggest almost complete relapse after 3-5 yr. The paucity of data provided by the weight-loss industry has been inadequate or inconclusive. Those who challenge the use of diet and exercise solely for weight control purposes base their position on the absence of weight-loss effectiveness data and on the presence of harmful effects of restrictive dieting. Any intervention strategy for the obese should be one that would promote the development of a healthy lifestyle. The outcome parameters used to evaluate the success of such an intervention should be specific to chronic disease risk and symptomatologies and not limited to medically ambiguous variables like body weight or body composition."

Methods for voluntary weight loss and control. NIH Technology Assessment Conference Panel.

A panel of experts convened by the National Institutes of Health determined that "In controlled settings, participants who remain in weight loss programs usually lose approximately 10% of their weight. However, one third to two thirds of the weight is regained within one year [after weight loss], and almost all is regained within five years."

Bacon L, Aphramor L: **Weight Science, Evaluating the Evidence for a Paradigm Shift**

"Consider the Women's Health Initiative, the largest and longest randomized, controlled dietary intervention clinical trial, designed to test the current recommendations. More than 20,000 women maintained a low-fat diet, reportedly reducing their calorie intake by an average of 360 calories per day and significantly increasing their activity. After almost eight years on this diet, there was almost no change in weight from starting point (a loss of 0.1 kg), and average waist circumference, which is a measure of abdominal fat, had *increased* (0.3 cm)"

So let's sum up here: Telling someone that they should lose weight to be healthier is telling them to do something nobody has proven is possible for a reason nobody has proven is valid.

It's ok though. If you want to be healthy, there is another option: Actually focusing at your health.

<u>Health at Every Size</u>

Health at Every Size is a health paradigm where the focus is put on health rather than body size as the measure of health. Writing that now makes it seem "face-palm" obvious, but I was so steeped in the thin=healthy diatribe that it took me a while to wrap my head around it.

There are many ways to practice Health at Every Size, my practice is built on the following:

There are healthy and unhealthy people of every shape and size.

Health is multi-dimensional and includes:

- Genetics
- Access to healthcare, including money, distance, time, hours of operation, and the ability to get a doctor who will give you appropriate care
- The ability to acquire, store and afford the kinds of foods that you want
- Access to safe movement options that you enjoy (where safe means both physically safe and emotionally safe including certainty that you won't be bullied)
- Stress
- Environment
- Behaviors, past and current

Health is never guaranteed, but the evidence suggests that practicing healthy behaviors gives us the best chance of being healthy--certainly a better chance than just trying to have a smaller body.

So that's how I live my life. I eat a healthy, balanced diet and, as a competitive dancer, I am extremely active. I have fantastic strength, stamina and flexibility, all of my metabolic measures are in the very healthy range (cholesterol, glucose, blood pressure, etc.), and my body is still fat.

Yet people tell me I can't be healthy doing those things and I would be much healthier if I:

Drink two thin chocolate beverages containing laxatives and eat one meal a day which is low fat and low carb.

Eat reconstituted soy protein five times a day and one meal of low fat protein and green vegetables.

Eat a certain number of calories (or "points") regardless of where they come from.

Eat a bacon double cheeseburger but hold the lettuce, tomato and bun.

Take pills, the side effects of which require a label that suggests I "wear dark pants and bring an extra pair to work."

Eat an extremely limited low calorie diet 6 days a week and binge on the 7th day.

Eat breakfast cereal four times a day with a meal of lean proteins and low carbs for dinner.

Eat a ton of cabbage soup and on Tuesday eat as many bananas as I want but nothing else.

What the...? The main difference between my diet and all the others appears to be that people make money selling those other diets and mine is what I think we would come to if we weren't being inundated with messages from the people making sixty billion dollars a year selling us snake oil. I can't believe how controversial it is to promote the idea of eating healthy, moving your body and letting it be whatever size it may be naturally, (I get death threats for doing exactly that) but I think that speaks more to the success of the diet company marketing machine than it does to anything bearing a resemblance to the realities of human health.

Shed Those Unhealthy Thoughts

Say I'm going to learn Spanish. My plan is to start by berating myself as often as possible for not already speaking Spanish. I'm going to hang up pictures of people who speak Spanish and every time I look at them I'm going to tell myself how much better they are than I am. As I learn Spanish I'll constantly focus on the things that are difficult for me and use my inner voice, which is now trained to berate me at every possible opportunity, to remind me I'm not good enough at speaking Spanish and probably never will be.

Sound like a good plan? How do you think it's going to go?

Then why do we do that when we try to get healthier?

Consider that if you want your body to be healthier, stronger, or more flexible you could start by appreciating where you are now. I'm guessing your heart is beating, you are breathing, and blinking. That's a nice place to start. Thank your body for that. Appreciate it for a minute. You don't even have to ask it; your body just breathes and blinks and beats your heart for you all day every day.

If you want to be stronger, how about starting by appreciating the strength you have now. Can you lift a gallon of milk? Great! Did you just move up from 5 lb to 10 lb dumbbells? Kick ass! Now what do you want to do?

Maybe stop comparing yourself to other people. Your body is your own. Nobody else has a body exactly like yours. That in itself is incredible. We're not chairs from IKEA; we are completely unique, one of a kind. I'm starting to sound a little bit "after school special" right now, but seriously, so many things in the world are mass-produced, yet you are a complete original. That's something truly special and worthy of appreciation.

Notice the messages that can seep into your subconscious. When you started to read the title of this section did you automatically think I was going to say "Shed those unhealthy pounds"? That's not accidental. The messages bombarding us about our bodies are often crafted to create fear and self-loathing. Then the message creator will try to make us believe that buying their product will cure the fear and self-loathing their message created.

I believe success breeds success, so anytime I have any little bit of success I do not hesitate to do a butt-shaking happy dance. If I accomplish this thing or that thing, it makes it that much easier to tackle the next goal on my path. If I fail, I remind myself this is a temporary state and promptly learn the lesson and forget about the rest as soon as possible. That works so much better for me than hating myself and reminding myself what I haven't accomplished yet.

Did you ever watch the movie "Cool Runnings"? It was loosely based on the first Jamaican Olympic bobsled Team. In it, one of the characters is asked what "Cool Runnings" means and he says it means "Peace be the journey." Since they are a bobsled team, I take that to mean not that things will be smooth, slow and easy, but that you can still be at peace through the difficult parts. Anytime we want to change or improve, it involves a journey; there's no getting around that. You can be happy or miserable on the way; that's your choice. For me it's definitely Cool Runnings! Peace be the journey…

Fitness and Fatness – One more round

Surprisingly often, people incorrectly assume (often out loud or in comments on my blog) that I "can't climb a flight of stairs without being winded" because I'm fat. But in the same breath, they say the only reason I can leg press 1,000 pounds or do a standing heel stretch is *because* I'm fat. What?

Of course, this doesn't make any sense – our strength, stamina and flexibility are the result of a combination of our genetics, access to movement options, information and professional assistance; and how much we work on each of them.

These statements are typically made by people who are acting like idiots and trying to diminish our accomplishments so they can hold onto their stereotypes and sense of superiority at all costs. I don't care so much about it when it comes at me, but I do worry that other people, who may not have had the opportunities to understand health that I have, will believe the oft-repeated but anatomically indefensible assertion that the only way to gain strength, stamina and flexibility is to lose weight.

We've talked a lot in this book about how intentional weight loss fails. Let's look at some ways movement succeeds:

"Groundbreaking work on fitness and weight has been done by [epidemiologist Steven] Blair and colleagues at the Cooper Institute. They have shown that the advantages of being fit are striking and that people can be fit even if they are fat … and thus have lowered risk of disease. A remarkable finding is that heavy people who are fit have lower risk than thin people who are unfit."
-Dr. Kelly Brownell, Director of the Yale Center for Eating and Weight Disorders, 2003

"We've studied this from many perspectives in women and in men and we get the same answer: It's not the obesity—it's the fitness."
-Steven Blair, P.E.D., Cooper Institute for Aerobics Research, 2004

"Active obese individuals actually have lower morbidity and mortality than normal weight individuals who are sedentary … the health risks of obesity are largely controlled if a person is physically active and physically fit."
-The President's Council on Physical Fitness and Sports, 2000

"This prospective follow-up study among middle-aged and elderly men and women indicates that obesity (as assessed by increased BMI) is not related to an increased risk of all-cause and CVD mortality, but low-level LTPA [leisure time physical activity] and a low level of perceived physical fitness and functional capability are … In conclusion, in contrast with our initial hypothesis, obesity was not found to be an independent predictor of mortality among middle-aged and elderly men and women. However, low-level LTPA seemed to predict and a low level of perceived physical fitness and functional capability predicted an increased risk of all-cause and CVD mortality among both men and women."
-*International Journal of Obesity Related Metabolic Disorders*, 2000

More and more evidence tells us the best thing we can do for our health is move our bodies 30 minutes a day, 5 days a week (for a great piece on this, search for 23 and 1/2 hours on YouTube by DocMikeEvans). As always, everybody gets to decide how much they want to prioritize their health and what path they want to take. However, when you're fat, especially if you've been fat for a while, even if you want to move there can be a lot of baggage and issues around exercise that stand in your way.

One of the heartbreaking things for me when I teach dance workshops, whether I'm teaching people recovering from eating disorders or a Health at Every Size Meet-up group, is the number of people who have never moved their body for any reason other than to punish themselves for eating and/or to try to change their body's size and shape.

I remember my years of trying to lose weight. I would work out all week and then feel like a failure if I didn't lose "enough" weight. I was told, incorrectly, that if my exercising didn't make me thin, it wouldn't make me healthy. But there is literally a mountain of evidence to contradict that. It appears exercise is the great equalizer. Fat people who exercise live longer than thin people who don't, and have virtually the same predicted lifespan as thin people who do exercise.

I'm not trying to tell you what to do; I'm just suggesting we take a look at some of the messages we get about exercise and then decide what we want to do.

Why do we not hear about the vast benefits of exercise? Maybe because it's not proven to lead to weight loss? In fact, while the diet industry spends billions of dollars on marketing and funding "scientific" studies and misleading the public into believing its solution works, nobody is pouring billions of dollars into the message that movement is likely to make you healthier even though it probably won't make you thinner.

When studies came out saying exercise did not lead to weight loss, a litany of "news" sources published reports that overlooked the benefits of exercise entirely and told people that they might be better off NOT exercising since it didn't help lose weight. What in fit fat hell are they doing?

The most egregious to me was a Time Magazine article which lost any modicum of credibility as far as I'm concerned by writing: "after you work out hard enough to convert, say, 10 lb. of fat to muscle — a major achievement…" A major achievement indeed since it's physically impossible. Muscle does not convert to fat. You gain or lose fat; you gain or lose muscle, they are two separate things. I get that this is stated a lot and that many people believe it, but how does someone who wants us to trust him as a health reporter make this mistake?

The ways in which this article gets science wrong are so numerous they would require an entire chapter, so I'll just leave it for now pointing out that the reports all mention study participants didn't lose weight, but they fail to discuss what health benefits participants may have received. Based on all the research available, we would expect to see improvements in one or more the following: blood glucose, blood pressure, triglycerides, insulin use by the body, cholesterol, strength, stamina, flexibility, and self-esteem.

But I mean, if it's not going to make my body smaller then why would I do it? (Sarcasm meter at a 10 out of 10 again.)

Plenty of people who develop heroin habits lose weight, but they don't experience increases in strength, stamina or flexibility as a result. People lose fat through liposuction, but they don't get any healthier for fitter as a result. I am ginormous but I have the strength, stamina and flexibility of a professional athlete. I think if you want to be healthier, it couldn't hurt and might help to find some form of movement you enjoy. The research says that 30 minutes (which can be broken up throughout the day) of moderate exercise, like walking, gardening, dancing around your living room, about five days a week is the number to shoot for but any is better than none if better health is your goal.

Athletic Physique, Dancer's Body, and Other Lies

My very thin friend called me crying. She had taken weeks to
work up the courage to go to a belly dance class only to be told
by the plus-sized belly dance instructor that she shouldn't bother
taking the class because she "doesn't have anything to shake". I
got the teacher's name and address, went to the studio and
helped change the instructor's perspective. I know just how my
friend felt - I, and many people my size, have been told we
shouldn't dance because we don't have a "dancer's body."

Dancer's body. Swimmer's Build. Athletic physique.

Complete, total and utter bullshit. All of it.

These ideas are constantly touted by two groups of people:

1. People who want to sell us something "Buy my
Taepilatyogalletboxing System and get that dancer's body
you've always wanted"

2. People who rely on feeling superior in order to feel okay
about themselves: "I have a dancer's body so it doesn't matter
how well you dance, you can't possibly be a dancer because you
don't have a dancer's body. I am therefore better than you and
so my fragile sense of self-esteem and exaggerated sense of self-
importance both remain intact."

Except nobody actually has the right to declare anything about
anybody else's body.

Do you dance? Do you want to? Then congratulations, you
have a dancer's body.

Do you swim? Do you want to? Then you have a swimmer's build. (Let's try to remember that everything from minnows to whales swims, you know what I'm saying?)

Are you an athlete? Do you want to be? Then you have an athletic physique.

People can try to tell us otherwise, but happily we get to decide if we're going to let people keep us from doing what we want to do because they are trying to sell us something or put us down to make themselves feel better about themselves. And we get to choose how we do it. Do we want to find a comfortable accepting environment (even if it's our living room)? Do we want to crash the party with our "non-traditional" bodies? It's all up to us.

Un-breaking Up with Exercise

Did you and exercise have a bad break-up? Was it because of dodge ball? Do you still have nightmares about your gym teacher's whistle? Did someone tell you exercise would lead to weight loss and when it didn't you quit because you figured it wasn't doing any good anyway? Or is not exercising your way to give a big 'ole Eff You to all the people who constantly tell you that you need to exercise?

If you are feeling like you and exercise could use some couples counseling, you are not alone. Here are my thoughts on how you and exercise might get back together and live happily ever after if you want:

The first thing is to consider letting go of whatever happened in the past. If you want health now, you probably have to forgive, or at least forget, your idiot gym teacher – unless you're cool with them affecting your current health.

If you're hoping for weight loss, you're probably barking up the wrong treadmill. Research tells us exercise will make us healthier but is unlikely to lead to weight loss, and even if it does, health and weight loss are both side effects of the behavior. Weight loss doesn't make people healthier, it just makes them smaller. So if you are looking at weight (instead of metabolic health markers and/or intrinsic messages such as how you feel,) you are likely to miss the actual benefits you receive from movement.

You may need to determine who you are doing this for. In my experience the problem with rebelling against people by being unhealthy is that we are the ones who suffer. The problem with doing healthy habits for other people is that we tend to resent them if we don't like the habits or don't get the results we want. Finally, decide what you are going to try first, set some reasonable expectations, and then decide what – if anything – you want to measure.

If you are looking for structure I highly recommend Jeanette DePatie at www.thefatchick.com, Jeanette has a book and a DVD that give a 12 week program. (For the record, Jeanette and I became friends after I started recommending her stuff, and I do not get paid to endorse her, I just think she's awesome.)

I always recommend figuring out what you want to try first in terms of exercise, then get a baseline and be totally okay with whatever it is. If you want to try walking, go for a walk. If you make it five minutes, that's awesome. Then set some kind of reasonable plan. Maybe your goal is five minutes a day five times a week with the goal of increasing to 10 minutes in a couple of weeks. Take it easy; you have your whole life to move your body, and you do not want to be the fittest person in traction.

Remember: You have nothing to punish yourself for and nothing to prove. This is a whole new thing, and this is the first day of it. Relax.

If you don't like the first thing you try, try something else. Try exercising with friends and alone to see what you like. Mix it up. Consider not planning. Set aside the time to do the exercise, but allow yourself to choose whatever appeals to you on the day. Remember you can break up the exercise into chunks – it doesn't have to happen all at once to get the benefits. Ten minutes in the morning, ten at lunch, ten after dinner is your thirty minutes. Walking from the back of the parking lot or up and down the stairs totally counts.

If you are one of those people who just doesn't like exercise, I feel your pain. As a dancer I often do stuff that I don't like. Flexibility is really important, for example, but I do not enjoy flexibility work. However, it's worth it to me to do it to meet my goals, so I try to cut down the misery as much as possible by listening to music I like or watching TV, and I just do it. I also find it helpful to remember that it's me and my body tackling flexibility, not me against my inflexible body.

In my opinion the absolute best thing you can possibly do is come to exercise on your own terms.

- If you find the word exercise triggering, then substitute something else – movement, working out, whatever.

- Celebrate every single victory. Walked two minutes more today than yesterday? Booty-shaking happy dance – rock on!

- Get the best equipment you can afford. If you are going to walk regularly, your body will thank you for having good supportive walking shoes.

- Stretch. It does wonders to prevent joint pain (much of which is from muscular imbalances or tightness pulling on the joints and has nothing to do with weight.)

- Consider adding a little strength training. More muscle will help you move that big body around and support your joint health (since the muscle will take the load and not the joints.)

- Consider adding Pilates. Core strength has been key for me and a lot of other fathletes I know.

- Go slow, and if you feel some discomfort, honor that and take it easy. Remember mixing up your workouts can help you avoid injuries due to repetitive motion.

- If you have access, water workouts are awesome, even done once in a while to give your body a break from walking or other higher impact activities.

- Decide what you want from this experience and create the entire experience to work just for you.

Exercise serves you, you do not serve exercise. You are the boss of your exercise underpants! Occupy your exercise underpants!

Guilt Does Not Burn Calories

In your last fitness class, when the teacher encouraged you to appreciate your body, what specific things came to mind?

I'll give you a minute to stop laughing. Fitness instructors who encourage you to appreciate your body for anything other than getting smaller are few and far between.

I am an aerobics class participant and instructor from way back. I did Step Aerobics on homemade steps it was first invented. I have literally taken thousands of group exercise classes and I can count on one hand the number of those classes that were taught from a positive perspective, where students were encouraged to be active for their health and to appreciate their bodies rather than hate their bodies and try to change their body size and shape.

All I remember from my exercise classes were statements about the horror of having body fat and vague assertions that "bikini season was coming."

I've noticed that a lot of fitness instructors seem to have the mistaken idea that they are somehow better than their students and that people who come to their class are unable to motivate themselves and thus need to be treated poorly, berated for not working hard enough, etc.

And don't think I wasn't guilty of the same things. When I taught aerobics I encouraged my students to bring outfits to class that were too small for them and hang them on the wall for motivation. I actually used the phrase, "If you don't squeeze it, nobody else will" while doing squats. I was 18 years old and convinced the only way to get people to work hard was through guilt, fear and shame.

Oh, how the tides have turned... my tides, anyway. These days, if a student asked I would suggest they donate the outfit that doesn't fit to Goodwill and go buy some clothes that they can love wearing now. I actively encourage students in my dance classes to appreciate their awesome bodies and everything those bodies are doing for them. I am certain that whether or not I squeeze it, someone else will.

Just for fun, I attended a step class and it was the same old stuff. Here are some of the instructor's greatest hits:

"Since you're just starting an exercise program be sure to take it slow, I wouldn't use a riser at all…" I replied in a calm, friendly matter, "Why would you think I'm just starting an exercise program?" She fumbled for a minute and then just sort of slowly backed away. Off to a rockin' start…

"Give me all you've got. Give a little extra for all the fat girls eating bon bons right now!" Okay, first, why is it always freaking bon bons? I'm a certified, bona fide, in-the-flesh fat girl and I'm not even sure what a bon bon is. Also, this seems vaguely like, "Eat your peas because children in [insert third world country] are starving." I don't believe ignoring my body's signals and working past its limitations will help sedentary people enjoy the benefits of exercise as much as it will lead to me being sedentary while I wait for my injuries to heal.

"Bikini season is here, and there's nothing worse than a muffin top!" Really? There's nothing worse? A muffin top is not cancer; let's not act like it is.

And my favorite…

wait for it…

"If you don't squeeze it, nobody will!" I laughed out loud at that one.

After class she asked me what I thought and I gently (no, seriously – I'm trying to have a teachable moment here, not throw a fit) gave her my feedback. "I liked the choreography and I got a good workout. I was put off right at the beginning by your assumption that I was just starting an exercise program, and I find I'm not very motivated by someone telling me to hate my body. Being fat, I certainly didn't appreciate your motivating the class by suggesting that they don't want to look like me. Out of curiosity, have you ever considered motivating students by encouraging them to appreciate their bodies and take care of them with healthy habits?" She literally laughed out loud and said "Nobody cares about being healthy; we all just want to be thin. You can say what you want but you wouldn't be exercising if you didn't want to lose all that fat." As I tried to control my rage before replying, she said she had to go and shut down future communication. Okie dokie.

I find it unconscionable to try to motivate people by convincing them they should hate the body they have now. As fitness instructors, we can do better, and as fitness class participants we should demand better.

If you are in a fitness class where your instructor encourages you to appreciate your body, consider thanking them!

If you're in a fitness class where you are encouraged to think of your body as flawed and ugly, or constantly told to be in terror of gaining weight, maybe it's time to reconsider your fitness environment or give the instructor some feedback.

Think of all of the thing things your body is doing for you to allow you to participate in class, and have a little gratitude. Your body is just awesome and deserves your love and devotion.

Won't Somebody PLEASE Think of the Joints?

You know - the joints that supposedly can't possible carry our weight. Except that they can and do. People who are 400 pounds complete marathons – our bodies are amazing and adaptive and that includes our ability to be fathletic. First they tell us that we need to exercise, and then they tell us our bodies can't take it. You gotta love a lose/lose scenario.

The claim that joint pain is caused by obesity sometimes goes with the claim that the human body "wasn't meant to carry [insert completely random number of] pounds." It also goes hand in hand with the VFHT, in this case taking advantage of the fact that bodies break down over time to say that if my joints do, it will be because of my fat.

There have been a few times in my life, at various weights, when I've had knee pain. When I was thinner doctors looked at things like muscle imbalances and tightness, and sure enough those were the (solvable) problems.

When I had knee problems a few years ago the only explanation offered to me by doctors was that I needed to lose weight. Because I had the luxury of knowing how they treat these issues with smaller people, I asked if thin people get joint problems. The doctor admitted that they do. I asked if thin people were told that weight loss was the only solution to their joint problems. Not catching on to where I was going he say "No, of course not – they are already thin". So I smiled politely and asked that try those interventions first.

While it seems to be convenient for doctors to blame everything that ever goes wrong in my life (seriously – obesity induced strep throat?) on my weight, I insist we exhaust other options first, and the other options always seem to work.

With this doctor, when I said I wanted to be treated like they treat thin people, I was told there was no point in treating any joint issues until I lost weight. What with the who now?

So I left the doctor's office and started working with a massage therapist and when we cleared up the tightness in my quads and IT band, the knee pain disappeared – the tight muscles and IT band were pulling the joint off center. Losing weight would have done NOTHING to help the actual issue – I would just have had knee pain in a smaller body. Later I started doing Pilates with Kate Wodash at The Mindful Body Center in Austin and I learned to correct my movement patterns to avoid the issues that caused the knee pain in the first place. I regularly do 75 full squat jumps (where you do a full squat, hands flat on the floor then jump up explosively) with no knee pain. Still 5'4", 284 pounds. Still have more fat (and more lean body mass) than most people.

In general I think a diagnosis of "fat" is just lazy medicine. If you are dealing with joint pain, and even if you are choosing to attempt weight loss as a solution, I highly suggest looking into other options that might help along the way. It may be that you need to strengthen the supporting muscles, or that your movement patterns have led to imbalance and you need to stretch the supporting muscles. Maybe you need to mix up your workout routine a little bit. Maybe a combination. Regardless, when joint pain is the problem, weight loss is not the only solution. Considering weight loss fails 95% of the time, I think it's worth it to give the other things a try.

My Feet Hurt Today

"My feet hurt today. My knee has a sharp pain when I bend it, my hip aches, and my left hamstring still hurts." I was I explaining this to my massage therapist. She was running late, so I had offered to talk in the lobby while her previous client was getting dressed to speed us along.

"I used to be big, too."

What?

I looked to my left and the gentleman, who I've never met before, is looking at me and whispering conspiratorially. I must have given him my patented "Oh, what in fat hell?!" look because he repeated himself in that same stage whisper "I used to be big, too." Undaunted by my heavy sigh and carefully cultivated utter-lack-of-interest face, he went on."The hardest thing to do is start," he informed me earnestly, "it's all about exercise. I know it's hard but you can just start walking five minutes a day, then increase to ten. I walk 45 minutes a day and I've lost 45 pounds". He executed a crescendo on the last sentence so that when he said "45 pounds" he was almost shouting and sticking out his chest with a level of pride I would personally reserve for the day that I cure cancer or climb Kilimanjaro.

I quelled my rage by reminding myself that he's a product of our culture. You can't swing a CNN news video without hitting an infomercial about how obese we all are and how it's causing everything from cancer to global warming.

He doesn't know I'm a professional dancer. Every other dancer I know, fat or skinny, complains about pain all the time. They joke that the injury never goes away, it just moves around. They are wrapped up, braced, iced, heated and rested. I don't want people to think I hurt because I'm fat, so I rarely admit to being in any kind of pain to people outside of my close circle.

He doesn't know my feet hurt because I've danced 27 hours this week and was choreographing until 4:00 am. He doesn't know my knee hurts because I increased my leg press to 30 reps at 420 lbs yesterday. He doesn't know my hip hurts because I have been jumping in the air and falling on it for a contemporary piece I'm working on, or that my hamstring hurts because I did a jump split without being properly warmed up. (Of course it was dumb, but that's hardly the point right now.) He doesn't know his entire workout wouldn't be a suitable warm-up for what I do. He's taught not to consider those as possibilities. I silently prepare for a teachable moment, starting with gently enlightening him as to some of the aforementioned things he didn't know about me.

It turns out he was about to know all those things, because my thin, quiet, massage therapist was opening a can of Whoop Ass. It all happened so fast that I couldn't completely follow it – suffice it to say she became some kind of Tasmanian Devil of Body Love. She started with a big "How DARE you"? There were middle bits about being closed-minded, uneducated and ignorant, a whole series of exasperated hand gestures, something about that if he and I started running he would be dead in a pile before I was warmed up, and ended with, "The next time you think about opening your mouth and spewing ignorant assumptions at one of my clients…don't!" His massage therapist, having heard this exchange as she walked around the corner, quickly called him back. As he went back she, also traditionally thin, admonished him for being rude, then walked back to me and apologized, saying that some people just don't understand the difference between health and weight and that she would give him a free education with his massage today.

First, I realized I am grateful beyond words for thin fat activists.

Second, I was reminded that I don't get to choose who I'm an example to, only what I'm an example of. I try to live my life out loud, and I keep finding that everything I hold back ends up holding me back. I'm a dancer. I'm in pain a lot - it's part of the deal. It comes with the territory. It's not because I'm fat, it's because I ask my body to do extraordinary things, and the only price it extracts is a little pain. Henceforth I will stop hiding any pain I'm in, and if people assume my pain is due to my size I'll have an opportunity for a teachable moment. Maybe somewhere another woman will be inspired to accept the pain that sometimes comes with athletic activity without feeling shame and believing it's because she's fat.

Third, I remembered how profoundly grateful I am to my body and the amazing practitioners who help keep it running.

So my feet hurt today, and that's just fine.

<u>Fatty Has Nothing to Prove and Nothing to Hide</u>

Society tries to hide fat healthy people. We don't fit into the idea that you can look at somebody and tell how healthy they are, we don't make the diet industry any money, and we won't just loathe ourselves like they want us to. I've found that when people are faced with a real live healthy fat person they often try to solve their newfound cognitive dissonance by challenging us to "Prove it." This is where I made a mistake, because I'm healthy and fat and athletic and a great fan of evidence, so I took up the challenge and started down a bad path. Let me tell you how this went and give you the chance to learn from my mistake:

Someone posted information about me on a listserv whose members were being reasonable and curious. They e-mailed me and asked me to state my numbers, so I posted my cholesterol, triglycerides, blood pressure, all of which were in the exceptionally healthy range. And they called me a liar and VFHTed me. I should have dropped out then, but I didn't.

One of these random strangers asked what I could do physically. So I posted pictures of my strength and flexibility.

They said that my ankle should have shattered 30 seconds after the first picture was taken, how could I hold my 284 pound body up on my toes like that? They said holding that 284 pound body up in an arch and doing suspended pull ups isn't hard. They said the reason I'm flexible must be because I'm all fat and no muscle. They asked why I didn't show something more athletic.

So I posted a picture of me leaping.

They said that if I did that twice I probably would shatter bones in my foot. (Never mind that I was doing this on concrete and that it was the 26th time because the photographer was working with a new lens.) My feet were fine. They asked couldn't I post anything where I was moving?

So I posted a dance video.

They said the dance I did was slow and that made it easy. (Dancers know this isn't true.) They said if I went any faster I would faint and be out of breath.

So I posted another, faster dance video.

They got mean. They called me a whale and a hippo. They said it doesn't matter because I'm still fat.

And there it was, staring me in the face. The truth. The reason "proving it" will never work. The only thing I had proven was that I could waste my time. Their core beliefs are that accomplishments only count if you're thin; therefore, since I'm fat, no amount of "proof" will ever be enough. I also realized that these are adults who resort to name calling and I was spending a lot of time trying to prove things to people for whom I have no more than basic human respect.

I've said before that I'm much more concerned with fat people realizing that they deserve respect than with other people realizing that fat people deserve respect. It turns out the same goes for posting pictures or videos or numbers. Don't like what I write? Don't believe me? I don't care. This isn't about you or for someone else. I'm done making that mistake.

The Other Role Model Problem

While people outside the HAES/SA community wring the hands and worry that successful fat people "promote obesity", within the community we have created our own role model problem." The Role Model Problem centers on whether or not a healthy fat person should speak about their health in terms of numbers. The concern is that a healthy fat person with good numbers might get sick, and then instead of being a role model they will become a cautionary tale. Also, proponents point out, health is not a barometer by which worth should be judged. Since everybody deserves to be treated with respect, there is no reason to talk about our numbers.

I completely understand this perspective. I see the merits and I respect everyone who chooses this. For these same reasons, I thought long and hard about putting my numbers out there, and I came to a different conclusion for myself.

I don't write or speak for the people who disagree with me. My work is for the people who are looking for an oasis of body love in a barren desert of body hate. We are bombarded with the idea that being fat is synonymous with being in poor health. We know that's untrue, and I think it's important to stand up to that stereotype.

Of course, I always want to be clear that health is multi-dimensional and that I don't consider health to be a moral, social, or personal obligation. I am very aware that my health isn't just because of my habits, it's also because of genetics, environment, access, and stress, just like everyone else's. Nobody's health is entirely within their control.

In her beautiful poem "Our Deepest Fear", Marianne Williamson points out that whether or not we realize it, shining our light lets other people know that they can shine theirs.

All any of us can do is choose to shine our light. Other people will chose insecurity, liberation, or something else as their reaction, but that's their choice, not our responsibility.

Society tries hard to hide people like me, and I don't really feel like helping them out. I believe healthy habits, while not a guarantee of health, are our best chance. If I get sick I won't start telling people, "Never mind, I was wrong eat crappy and never exercise." Elite athletes drop dead of heart attacks and get cancer, yet they don't lose their status as athletes who lived a healthy lifestyle. There is a tremendous double standard when fat athletes who get sick lose their status, and I simply refuse to buy into it.

We're all going to die eventually, and whether my health is ended by a fast-moving bus, old age, or alien abduction, someone will be standing around saying that it was because I was fat. So what? I'm not at all concerned with what these people think. I'm also much less concerned with being a "good role model" than I am with being authentically me. I feel good when I look for things to celebrate about my body instead of things to change or hate or hide. Right now those things include excellent numbers and I will not let fear of my inevitable death stop me from celebrating my body as it is, continuing pursuing things that may me feel good, and bucking a ridiculous unsupported stereotype every single chance I get.

My journey is about refusing to be hidden by society. This is because fat people deserve to see themselves represented as more than just a headless picture carrying a fast food bag and I can help with that. When it comes to fathleticism, there are fat people of all stripes – some are couch potatoes, some are active, some are hardcore athletes. Lots of us are healthy and happy. This is about showing an example of that.

Raising Our Physical Voices

As you may have noticed, I'm very vocal about being a fat dancer. I bring up my size. Often, someone asks me why – why do I have to be so "militant" about being fat? If nobody else is bringing it up, why do I feel the need to do it, especially when it makes people so uncomfortable. Here's why:

In my second year dancing competitively my waltz gown was a beautiful crushed velvet dress with spaghetti straps that I loved, and I always got compliments when I wore it. At the end of a competition, a judge named Cindy caught me at the elevators and told me that she "couldn't stand to look at me." I did a quick calculation (go off on her or be classy?). I chose classy and responded flatly "okay." She told me four more times that she couldn't stand to look at me. I just kept saying "okay," with no emotion. She kept getting louder and angrier. I kept saying "okay." She wagged her finger in my face, as her own face got red and she raised her voice "You have NO BUSINESS wearing spaghetti straps!" I said "okay." (Though I almost laughed at how ridiculous it was for her to get this emotional about my spaghetti straps.)

She pivoted, saying "You're such a beautiful dancer, but with your arms uncovered like that I couldn't stand to look at you." I made the (very difficult) decision to continue be classy and said, "In truth, I probably won't choose to change the dress, but I appreciate that you took the time to tell me it's such a problem for you." It was so clear to me in that moment that Cindy was trying to push her body image issues on me, and that I didn't have to accept them.

For a lot of my life, I've been an "exception," and I hear the same thing from a lot of my large friends. People say things to us like,

"I'm not attracted to big women, except you."

"I would never take a class from a plus-sized aerobics instructor, except you."

"I think of all big people are lazy, except you."

Being the exception means that, instead of taking a hard look at their prejudice, someone hangs onto it by sticking us in the "exception" category. That's not okay. I'm not interested in being the exception to stereotypes, I'm interested in obliterating stereotypes.

It's been said that dancing gives you a physical voice, and I agree. But it's not just dancing that provides a physical voice; it's all physical activities, including the act of just *being* in this culture. When people discount us as non-physical beings or as unworthy of being looked at because we're fat, they are trying to silence our physical voice. When Cindy told me that I should hide my arms because they were just too disgusting to be looked at, she was trying to silence my physical voice.

The reason that I bring up my size a lot when other people would like to pretend I'm "normal," and the reason I don't want to be the exception, is that when any of us claims a physical voice, they claim it for all of us. When we stand up for ourselves and raise our physical voices, we start to change perceptions, change prejudices, and make a difference in the world.

Life in the Fat Lane

So what can we do to live our happiest possible lives in the fat lane?

Yes, It's Okay to Be Fat

I want to talk about the idea that it's not ok to be fat, whether it's because of "health reasons", or aesthetic reasons, or the costs of being fat or whatever other reasons people come up with.

It doesn't matter how fat someone is, or why they are that fat, or what the outcomes of being that fat may or may not be. That person deserves to be treated with respect and it is completely ok for them to be that size. Yes, even if they weigh 2000 pounds. Yes even if you think their weight is "their fault." Yes, even if you would never ever want to be that fat. Yes, even if you can't understand how they live. Yes, even if they have problems that can be correlated with being fat. Yes, even if they have problems that can be causally related to being fat. Yes, even if studies show that they cost society more. Yes, even if they actually cost society more. It is totally, completely 100% ok for someone to be fat. Nobody needs anyone's encouragement, justification or permission to live in their body. Period. This is true whether or not it is possible to achieve permanent weight loss – it is a matter of civil rights.

It is wrong to find a group of people who are identifiable based on how they look, calculate their supposed cost on society, decide that the world would be cheaper without them, and then declare war and attempt to rid the world of them.

We have got to get this together as a community because there is a war actively being waged against fat people and every time we say "I'm not sure if it's ok to be fat" regardless of our reasons or intentions, we are fighting on the wrong side and we are making more fat people into casualties. It does not matter if you are fat or thin, if you're happy with your weight or if you are trying to change it – we have to stop asking whether or not fat people have the right to exist, and start demanding the right to life, liberty and the pursuit of happiness for people of every size – which includes the right to live my life, in our bodies, without having the government and private interests waging a war against us because of how we look.

Other people's body size is not anybody else's business. If we are interested in other people's health then I think that the only appropriate thing to do is work for access – ensuring that people have access to the foods that they would choose to eat, safe movement options that they would choose (which means both physically safe and mentally safe – so someone can walk around their gym in a bathing suit with no fear of negative comments etc.), affordable evidence-based health care, and true information. Then everyone gets to make their own decisions.

Each person is allowed to choose to attempt weight loss, that is their decision. Each person is also allowed to choose NOT to attempt weight loss. One person's decision to attempt weight loss does not invalidate another person's decision to live in a fat body.

People get to prioritize their own health. That means that they are allowed to drink like fish, jump out of helicopters wearing skis, be a cast member of Jackass, take stressful jobs, not get enough sleep, eat what they choose, be sedentary etc. at whatever weight they happen to be. Let's not forget that there are people of various weights who have the same diet and exercise routine, and people of the same weight who have very different diet and exercise routines. Acting as if all fat people engage in unhealthy behaviors and are unhealthy, and all thin people engage in healthy habits and are healthy is not supported by the evidence. It is stereotyping and bigotry, pure and simple.

We have every right to exist in the body we have now. Just so there is no confusion, I am saying that it is totally, entirely, completely ok to be fat.

Build a Good Relationship with Your Body

Growing up as an athlete I was told over and over again that my body was a limitation to be overcome and that I needed to have the mental toughness to move past the pain. It didn't come naturally at first – I seemed to have an innate sense that my body deserved better than that. But at some point I turned a corner and got really good at ignoring my body.

I worked through stress fractures, an IT band so tight it felt like it was going to rip in half, pulled muscles, sprains, strains, jammed fingers, knee injuries, and a host of other issues. I ignored my body when it asked for food and hydration and I scoffed at it when it asked for rest. I became a compulsive exerciser, and I started to look down on my body even more. I didn't give it what it needed and pushed it to first reasonable and then unreasonable limits. When my body finally bent or broke under the strain, I treated it with contempt. I believed my body was just a "meat sack," a collection of muscles and bones that were trying to limit what I could do. I believed my mind had to be stronger than my body, and I felt triumphant when I ignored my body's signals and "pushed through."

If I had an acquaintance who treated me the way I treated my body all those years, I would never speak to them again. In fact, I would never have let that kind of behavior go on so long. But through all of this my body stuck with me. Even though I wasn't giving it the food, hydration, or rest it needed, my body continued to support me. It never gave up on me. If my body could talk, all it would have said for years was either, "Will you please just give me what I need to do my job here?" Or, "For the love of all that's holy, can we please take a nap?!" But I wouldn't have listened.

I'm not saying you should never push your body; I've danced through plenty of injuries. What I'm suggested is that you treat your body like you would treat a friend. I can't even count the things my best friend has done for me, even though he didn't want to, because he's my best friend and he loves me and I asked. It's the same with my body. We have conversations:

Me: "Hey, body, those are some awesome four-inch heels. They'd go great with our blue and white dress. We could totally rock those."

Body: "Are you freaking kidding me? Do you know how hard our workout regimen is? Give me a break and go for the flats, please!"

Me: "Fair point. Flats it is".

Or this one:

Me: "Hey, body, I know I sprained our ankle yesterday being stupid, but I have a performance tonight and I'd really like to do it. Will you push through it with me if I promise to give you lots of ice and see the acupuncturist tomorrow?"

Body: "Yup, I'll help you out, but can we please take a couple of days off after the performance?"

Me: "Absolutely; thanks a bunch!"

Like any relationship, my body and I have to keep up the communication, but we've come a long way since our days of giving each other the silent treatment, and it's getting better all the time.

Community

One of the most important things for me is to have a community of people who are also into Size Acceptance and Health at Every Size.

Let me clarify the difference between the two one more time because it can get really confusing. Size Acceptance is the basic concept that every body of every size deserves to be treated with respect. I believe that Size Acceptance is a civil rights issue and that everyone should be for Size Acceptance, whether they are fat or thin, trying to lose weight or focusing on health separate from weight. Civil rights are not up for debate or a vote. We all have the right to life, liberty and the pursuit of happiness in the body that we have right now.

Health at Every Size is a health practice that is based upon focusing on healthy habits instead of weight – it's a new paradigm for health in which we stop using weight as a middleman and just focus on health.

If you're looking to meet other members of this community, there are great organizations like:

The Fit Fatties Forum – a free forum for people who want to talk about fitness from a Health at Every Size Perspective. There's a photo and video gallery, groups for newbies, oldbies, runners, belly dancers and more, discussions, and you can even ask your questions to an expert on the Ask a Fit Fatty Section. www.fitfatties.com

NAAFA – The National Association for the Advancement of Fat Acceptance (www.naafa.org).

ASDAH – The Association for Size Diversity and Health (www.sizediversityandhealth.org)

If you are online you can find all kinds of communities based around different principles. There are online forums, Facebook communities, and the fatosphere. If you go to my blog (www.danceswithfat.org) and check out the "Blogs I Love" page, you'll find some places to start exploring. Get involved with the blogs you like, comment, and friend the blogger on Facebook and Twitter.

Wherever you are in your journey with your body, it really helps to get some supportive community around you.

Activism

Doing some activism can really help you feel empowered. I think one of the hardest things about being an activist is people who feel like you have to live up to their expectations or decisions. It happened to me recently on my blog when a reader suggested that I post a food log. I said:

"No. I don't try to prove things to anybody anymore. I understand that you are well-intentioned and where you're coming from with this, but I'm not going to do it. I'll post my food log and then I'll have to deal with 1,000 comments and e-mails where people call me a liar, or tell me what I SHOULD be eating to lose weight, or offer to let me try their weight loss plan for free etc. I don't feel like dealing with it, and I don't owe anyone an explanation."

A reader named Barbara made the following comment in response:

"Ragen is an Activist. And unfortunately being an activist has to come with a certain amount of disclosure. You can't say, "Take my word for it."You can't say, "I am a fit, healthy, proud fat person who has nothing to hide and wants to share with the world that you can be fat and healthy" and then say, "Nobody will believe me if I put the information out there, so I'm not going to." You either believe that you are helping the cause, or you believe there is no changing people's minds and you are wasting your time."

Barbara is well-intentioned, but from my perspective she doesn't know much about being an activist and is way too into telling me what I should and shouldn't do. I think the most egregious issue with this is the phrase:

"…an activist has to…"

Personally, I don't feel those words should be put together in that order, ever. There was room for Malcolm X and Martin Luther King, Jr., Harvey Milk and Larry Kramer, Gloria

Steinem and Betty Ford. I am **IN NO WAY** comparing myself to any of these people, but they are all heroes of mine in one way or another and they had very different styles of activism, so I feel comfortable that there's room for fat activists who post food logs and for those of us who do not.

In fact, I think this is particularly true for fat activists. When we live in a world that constantly pummels us with messages that we are not healthy, not attractive, and not worthy of love, just getting out of bed in the morning and not hating ourselves is a revolutionary act. When so many fat people think they deserve to be shamed and stigmatized, standing up for our basic rights to be treated with respect and dignity constitutes activism, no food log required.

If it seems like I'm picking on Barbara, I'm not. I believe that she had the best of intentions. Her comments are representative of things I hear all the time from lots of people – what I'm obligated to do and who I'm obligated to be so I can meet their definition of an activist. For me, activism is about what we want to be and how we want to be it, not about trying to fit our picture into someone else's frame.

You be the boss of your fat activist underpants, and I'll be the boss of mine. I think we could use a whole lot more fat activism of all kinds and a whole lot less people telling us how we have to do it.

Be a Size Acceptance Activist Without Leaving the House

1. Support Size Acceptance

You deserve to be treated well right now. You deserve respect, and you have the right to life, liberty and the pursuit of happiness. Right now. In the body in which you currently reside.

Even if you want to eat differently or move more or whatever, I'm asking that you consider the possibility that your body is amazing and deserving of love and respect right this minute. Remember that no matter what your body looks like you are the standard of beauty in some culture somewhere. Beauty is arbitrary. Consider that the cure for social stigma is not weight loss, it's ending social stigma.

People have the right to choose how highly to prioritize their health and what path of health to take. It doesn't matter what you are doing or what you think other people should do. This is a civil rights issue. Even if you are choosing to diet to lose weight, even if you believe that's the only correct path to health. Size Acceptance gives you the right to choose that path just as it gives me the right to choose Health at Every Size and someone else the right to choose to be sedentary. Bodies are not a barometer upon which we should judge health, value, intelligence or anything else. Don't make assumptions or say nasty things about fat people. Don't make assumptions or say nasty things about thin people (especially if you're fat – the road to self-esteem and civil rights is not paved with hypocrisy). Every body deserves respect.

2. Come out as fat and happy

Harvey Milk is a huge hero of mine. He was the first openly gay man to be elected to a major public office. In my favorite of his speeches he said:

"Without hope the us's give up. I know that you can't live on hope alone, but without it, life is not worth living. And you, and you, and you, and you have got to give them hope."

One of Harvey Milk's main political tools was getting people to come out of the closet. The more out gay people someone knows, the more likely they are to see us GLBT people as humans, deserving of equal rights. Obviously there's no need for us to come out as fat, but there is another coming out that we can do. We can come out as fat *and* happy. Like this

"My name is Ragen Chastain and I am fat and happy. I love my life and I love my body. I eat to nourish my body a lot of the time, and sometimes I eat because I like orange sherbet. I went to the gym tonight for the pure joy of moving my body and I didn't even consider weighing myself because I don't care. If you don't like my body and/or want to make unsolicited suggestions about how I should treat it, then may I suggest you practice the ancient art of looking in another direction while keeping your mouth shut."

Sincerely,

~Ragen Chastain
Happy Fatty

3. Challenge Headless Fatty Images

I have had enough of pictures of fatties without heads being used to represent everything from greed to laziness to a supposed health crisis. Pictures of headless fatties– who were typically not compensated or asked for their permission – litter the internet. Our bodies are freely used for whatever the negative metaphor, comparison, or representation of the day is, not to mention to represent fat people in general. These pictures take away everything that is human about us and make us into a fat torso carrying a fast food bag. As if we have no feelings about seeing people who look like us constantly used to represent everything bad in the world. As if those feelings aren't important.

People don't take care of things if they don't think are worthy of care, so I consider the use of headless fatty pictures – which are designed to show fat bodies as shameful and bad – to be detrimental to public health.

Our bodies are not someone's to photograph and throw all over the Internet as a metaphor for anything. We are PEOPLE, these are our BODIES, and EVERY BODY deserves respect.

Every time you see a picture of a headless fatty on the Internet leave a comment like "No More Headless Fatties – Every Body Deserves Respect!" If you want to take it one step further send an e-mail to the source of the story – tell them your personal story. Let's teach people that this behavior isn't okay. This kind of activism can reframe this issue. Now, instead of feeling angry or hurt or ashamed when we see a headless fatty picture, we can look at it as a chance to educate people and stand up for ourselves.

4. Support Activism

Support organizations that support Size Activism by joining them, volunteering, and spreading the word about them among your community. Buy books from your favorite fat activists for full price instead of buying a used copy that won't pay them the royalty that they deserve. Send an e-mail to your favorite activists and bloggers and tell them that you like what they do, and how they have helped you. Trust me, on days when I get put on some fat hate thread and get 150 death threats, it can completely turn my day around to get one e-mail from someone telling me that my work inspired them or helped them through something.

5. Commit Public Displays of Fatness

A war against obesity is a war against obese people. And so the bodies that we live in 100% of the time have become political. No longer are we simply venturing out of our houses; we are committing Public Displays of Fatness:

EWF: Eating While Fat

Any time you eat in public when you're fat you risk having people comment to you. Things that have happened to me:

Eating a burger and fries: A perfect stranger says, "This is why you're fat." I responded, "You are way out of line and you don't know what you're talking about. How dare you? Move on."

Eating a salad: A perfect stranger says, "Good for you for working on it, but you should skip the cheese next time." I respond, "You are way out of line and you don't know what you're talking about. How dare you? Move on."

Either way, because I'm fat and have the "nerve" to eat in public, people feel they are justified in commenting if my food choice doesn't pass their test for what a fatty should eat, or they feel they are doing me a favor by encouraging what they assume must be an attempt to change the size and shape of my body, rather than just eat a tasty salad.

Reclaim your right to eat whatever the hell you want in public. Enjoy your food and tell people that if they're looking for their beeswax, they won't find it on your plate.

WWF: Working out While Fat

Picture this. I am at the gym doing HIIT (High Intensity Interval Training). I'm working as hard as I can, tracking my heart rate and my interval time. The person who has been walking on the machine next to me reading a magazine steps down and, before she leaves, says, "Good for you for starting an exercise program! Stick to it and you'll lose the weight." Now, I have no problem with someone walking on a treadmill reading a magazine – especially if they enjoy it. But I do have a problem with someone who has watched my intense cardio routine feeling comfortable making an assumption OUT LOUD, TO ME that I'm a beginner exerciser.

This is a really important one because fat people are constantly given the message that we are lazy and don't exercise, and those of us who are athletes get hidden away because showing us in a positive light would be "promoting obesity." So every time we are athletic in public it's a Big Deal. It's flipping the bird to all of those people who say that we don't or can't move our bodies, but more importantly it's giving fat people who hate their bodies because they don't think there is another option – a opportunity to see a different path: that we can love and move our bodies at any size.

DFA: Displays of Fat Affection

Remember when that idiot Marie Claire blogger said, "I think I'd be grossed out if I had to watch two characters with rolls and rolls of fat kissing each other, because I'd be grossed out if I had to watch them doing anything." That's real. That's something that a blogger for a major women's magazine website felt comfortable publishing online, under her real name. And her editors let it through.

If you are in a relationship and you are comfortable, I think being public about it is awesome. Again, it models another option for those fat people who've bought the war on obesity line that they are unattractive and unlovable because of their weight.

FIP: Fat in Public

This covers all the rest of the time. I'm always fat, but being fat in public can bring on anything from a car full of high school boys making mooing sounds to a well dressed gentleman lecturing me about how I'm costing him insurance money.

So what's to be done? If we want change, I think the first step is really looking at the culture that we live in, and the second step is choosing not to participate in that culture. Then take some actions:

Stop body snarking (and that includes people of all sizes). There is no reason in the world that you need to speak negatively about someone else's body. You are better than that.

Discourage other people from body snarking, or at least stop participating in the conversations and walk away.

Speak up about the difference between weight and health.

Actively seek out pictures that aren't the single standard of beauty that gets shoved down our throats by the media. Try fitfatties.com, the Fat Athletes group on Flickr, or www.adipositivity.com for a start

Even if you personally believe that obese people are lazy, unattractive drains on society or that losing weight is just a matter of calories in/calories out or whatever, consider the effect of your words and then consider keeping them to yourself. You can't make someone hate themselves healthy and I assure you that the person you are about to talk to has already heard what you are going to say. You are not The Fatty Whisperer, walk away.

Consider approaching your body from a place of care and appreciation.Consider spending the money that you would spend on diet programs on other self-care...get some massages, take classes that you've always wanted to take, buy a bike, hire a chef to prepare a delicious meal that will nurture your body, take a trip to a spa, buy amazing foods, whatever makes your body feel great.

Understand that almost everyone in our society is hurting because of ceaseless body shame and stigma. Even that person who you might think has "everything" – the perfect body, the perfect face - may be living his or her life in terror of losing it all. Look for ways to support other people and lift them up. I saw a woman at the bank with beautiful long, curly silver hair (exactly the kind of hair I plan to have someday). I told her that I thought her hair was awesome and she started crying. CRYING. At. The. Bank. She hugged me and told me that her friends said that you can't have long gray hair and that she should cut it. What the eff, people!? We can do better.

Commit the absolutely revolutionary act of loving yourself and your body right this second. Even if you want to change its shape and size, consider recognizing all of the amazing stuff that your body does for you and choosing to love it no matter what.

Now if you'll excuse me, I'm going to go EWF, then head to the gym for a little WWF, hopefully avoid a HFP, and then see if I can't get involved in a DFA. After that I think I'll just be FIP for a while.

I believe that in my lifetime I'll know what it's like to live in my body, in this culture, without constant societal stigmatization. But even if that doesn't happen, I believe in doing whatever I can to move us as far down the path as possible in the time that I have.

Stand Your Ground – Won't Back Down

One of the most frequently asked questions I get from blog readers is: "How do you explain to someone who doesn't believe in Health at Every Size that they are wrong?"

The short answer for me is that I probably don't. It can be extremely frustrating when other people don't respect our decisions about our personal health, but other people have a right to their opinions just as we have a right to ours. I can't argue that my choices are unlimited while simultaneously arguing to limit someone else's choices. I like dialog, but it's very difficult to have a discussion with someone who has stuck their fingers in their ears and is yelling, "LA LA LA LA LA!" So I think that it comes down to our right to decide how people treat us. Choosing to opt out of the diet culture can elicit a strong reaction for one of several reasons:

Good Cop: People are genuinely concerned

We are exposed to thousands and thousands of thin = healthy messages every day. Many of us, upon a thorough review of the evidence, have concluded that this information is erroneous. Other people haven't done the research, or they looked at the evidence and drew a different conclusion. They are genuinely worried about our health.

Bad Cop: Jealousy/Envy/Threat/Immaturity

Unfortunately for some people, their bodies made it out of Junior High School but their brains were left behind. Some have bought into the diet culture wholesale, and the fact that we haven't bothers them. Some people need to convince other people that they are right in order to feel good about their own decisions. Some people need to feel superior. Some people can only feel good about themselves when they are putting someone else down.

No matter why they are acting like this, you can choose how you are treated. I heard the lyric "way too up to back down" today and it captured exactly how I feel. When I was dieting, trying desperately to be thin so that I could be healthy, I ended up being anything but healthy – physically or mentally. Now I enjoy health without obsessing about food and exercise. I'm way too up to back down on this issue. Unless someone has some serious evidence to present to me, I'm not interested. So what do you say to people who are giving you an "everybody knows" answer?

Discussion

If the person is important to you, consider a conversation. Decide ahead of time what you want. Are you open to a discussion? If so, what are the ground rules? You get to decide. Maybe this is something that you and this person just won't talk about. If they're unwilling to comply with your wishes, you need to know what you're going to do. Are you prepared to walk away? Can you listen to these things from them in the future and take what they have with a grain of salt?

Disconnection

Typically I'm a fan of discussion but I've come to realize that sometimes the person in question just isn't worth the trouble. If that's the case, you might want to consider disconnecting from them and moving on. You can still be pleasant, just pull away quietly. Do it with class but consider the idea that you have a finite amount of time and attention to give, you get to choose who you give it to, and some people do not deserve your time and energy.

Confrontation

You can certainly go with the yelling, screaming approach. In my experience – and I don't think this is fair, it's just been my experience – becoming emotional often makes my argument seem weak and makes me feel powerless in the situation. Your mileage may vary, so if it feels good to get it out, then by all means do what you want.

Regardless of what you do, I highly recommend building a network of people who will support you. If you can't do it in person, then start looking online. Find a group who you can trust; being there for each other is incredibly helpful.

Mantras for Fatty Sanity

I have suffered a lot because I'm obese, but I've never suffered from obesity. My suffering comes from living in a society that says that the way to end the shame, stigma, humiliation and incompetent healthcare that we have to deal with is for us to lose weight. I suffer from living in a society where I'm the subject of a witch hunt but instead of dunking me in the river they put me on a scale. That suffering has nothing to do with my actual body size and everything to do with people refusing to acknowledge that the cure for social stigma is not weight loss.

Living in this society with your health, sanity and sense of humor intact can be tough. I have developed some strategies that help me:

Mantras:

Whenever I'm on the internet reading the latest ridiculous fat bashing articles or I'm overwhelmed by the amount of sheer jackassery in a comment, I have a little mantra that I say (typically to myself and not out loud for reasons that are about to become obvious).

The world is fucked up. I'm fine.

If fuck is not your second favorite f word, feel free to substitute whatever works for you. This little mantra has saved me on many occasions. Sometimes I add "and I'm doing something about it" to the end.

Another one that I've given to people who do feel like they want to lose weight but are having trouble get their head above the fat shame waters is:

Nobody deserves to be treated this way.

It really doesn't matter what your habits are or were, or what size your body is. Nobody deserves to be treated the way that fat people are treated in our society. Especially when the same people who are slamming us certainly have their own vices, but as long as they keep them hidden they feel like they can make themselves feel better by making fat people feel bad. No more.

Remember that dance judge who cornered me against the elevator and kept telling me that she couldn't stand to look at me because I was wearing spaghetti straps. I decided to keep responding by flatly saying "okay" while she got more and more emotional. It became very clear that she wanted to pass her body image issues on to me. While I'm a fan of presents, this is a crappy gag gift that I don't want. For situations like these I often think to myself

These are your issues, and I don't want them. You can keep them.

It helps keep me centered and reminds me that I don't look at myself through other people's eyes and I don't measure myself by other people's rulers anymore. I tried doing that, it was horrible, I don't need to go back to that place.

What If I'm Wrong?

In science, we always have to leave the possibility that we might be wrong, and any scientist who doesn't freely say that they could be wrong is no kind of scientist. There were times in our history when the best science "proved" that the Earth was flat and the sun revolved around it, that giving pregnant women thalidomide was a good idea, and that heroin was a fantastic cough suppressant.

I've examined a lot of scientific evidence about weight and health, and I've decided that a preponderance of the evidence points to a Health at Every Size approach. There's the fact that no study on weight loss has ever been successful, and that over 95% of everyone who diets fails. Dr. Linda Bacon, Paul Campos, Dr. Deb Burgard, and Dr. Jon Robinson and a host of other experts and the information they've shared have led me to what I believe is a sound scientific decision that healthy behaviors are more likely to lead to a healthy body than the lifelong pursuit of a specific height-to-weight ratio.

But just as I believe all of those people pushing the idea the thin = healthy are wrong, I know that I, too, might be wrong. It's possible that I would live a longer life if I just kept trying diet after diet in the hopes that I would find one for which I am in the magical 5% who can achieve weight loss.

I also realize that, even if I'm not wrong, the drivel that passes for science these days correlationally relates everything you can die from to being fat (including swine flu. Seriously…swine flu.) I'm pretty sure that if I died because a giant flock of geese dropped a piano on my head, the report from the coroner would say that I died of fatness.

I digress. I saw a great interview with Will Smith, of whom I have long been a fan, in which he said, "You have to say, This is what I believe, and I'm willing to die for it. Period. It's that simple. You have to be willing to die for the truth." I agree with him 100%.

Here is what I think is true:

While many things have been correlated to obesity (using some very questionable science), almost nothing has been successfully causally related (despite a staggering number of attempts).

Even if they could prove that obesity caused health problems, there isn't a single thing that has been proven to succeed at creating long term weight loss (despite even more numerous attempts). So there is no "cure".

The cycle (yo-yo) dieting that occurs when the vast majority of people fail at one diet and then move on to the next is being shown to be more harmful than just being fat

I am the picture of health by every measure in the world EXCEPT a measure by which people look at me and judge my health based on nothing more than the size of my body.

But what if I'm wrong?

There is a 100% chance that I'm going to die, so I don't think that's what's important. I think what's important is how I live. I spent almost all of my childhood, all of my teens and a decent chunk of my 20s buying into the diet industry's version of truth, and I was sick and miserable and still fat. I know people who are in their 40s, 50s, 60s and older still living a life of guilt, shame and weight obsession, crippled by their low self-esteem because they choose to buy into the diet culture and believe that they aren't worthy until they are thin which they have spent their whole lives failing at.

I live a life of health and joy, people tell me that I help them, and if I die immediately after this book goes to print, I will be happy and satisfied with the life I gave. I seriously doubt that I'm going to die of fatness, but if I'm wrong, the truth is that when I was trying to be thin my life was miserable, and I wouldn't want three or five extra years of that. If I am wrong then I chose to live a joyful, short life. But I think I'll stick around to see if they are still VFHTing me when I'm 102.

Now it's your turn to decide.